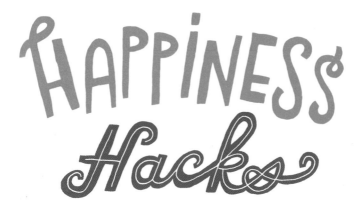

HAPPINESS
Hacks

Also by Alex Palmer

The Santa Claus Man: The Rise and Fall of a Jazz Age Con Man and the Invention of Christmas in New York

Weird-o-Pedia: The Ultimate Book of Surprising, Strange, and Incredibly Bizarre Facts About (Supposedly) Ordinary Things

Alternative Facts: 200 Incredible, Absolutely True(-ish) Stories

Literary Miscellany: Everything You Always Wanted to Know About Literature

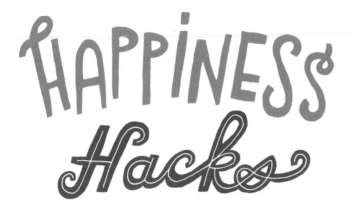

HAPPINESS
Hacks

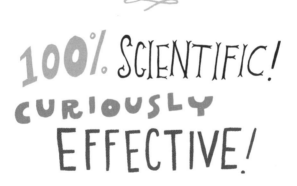

100% SCIENTIFIC!
CURIOUSLY
EFFECTIVE!

ALEX PALMER

THE EXPERIMENT

NEW YORK

The Experiment, LLC | 220 East 23rd Street, Suite 600 | New York, NY 10010-4658
theexperimentpublishing.com

This book contains the opinions and ideas of its author. It is intended to provide helpful and informative material on the subjects addressed in the book. It is sold with the understanding that the author and publisher are not engaged in rendering medical, health, or any other kind of personal professional services in the book. The author and publisher specifically disclaim all responsibility for any liability, loss, or risk—personal or otherwise—that is incurred as a consequence, directly or indirectly, of the use and application of any of the contents of this book.

Many of the designations used by manufacturers and sellers to distinguish their products are claimed as trademarks. Where those designations appear in this book and The Experiment was aware of a trademark claim, the designations have been capitalized.

The Experiment's books are available at special discounts when purchased in bulk for premiums and sales promotions as well as for fund-raising or educational use. For details, contact us at info@theexperimentpublishing.com.

Library of Congress Cataloging-in-Publication Data

Names: Palmer, Alex, 1981- author.
Title: Happiness hacks : 100% scientific! curiously effective! / by Alex
  Palmer.
Description: New York, NY : Experiment, [2018] | Includes bibliographical
  references.
Identifiers: LCCN 2018000505 (print) | LCCN 2018006836 (ebook) | ISBN
  9781615194438 (ebook) | ISBN 9781615194421 (pbk.)
Subjects: LCSH: Happiness. | Self-actualization (Psychology)
Classification: LCC BF575.H27 (ebook) | LCC BF575.H27 P356 2018 (print) | DDC
  158--dc23
LC record available at https://lccn.loc.gov/2018000505

ISBN 978-1-61519-442-1
Ebook ISBN 978-1-61519-443-8

Cover and text design by Sarah Smith
Author photograph by Greg Naeseth

Manufactured in the China

First printing May 2018
10 9 8 7 6 5 4 3 2 1

CONTENTS

1: What Is Happiness?... 7

2: Happy at Work 13

3: Happy at Play 31

4: Happy in Love.. 50

5: Happy at Home 66

6: Happy in Friendship.. 82

7: Happy in Health... 101

8: High-Tech Happiness 119

9: Finding Your Happy Place.................................... 135

10: The Downside of Happiness................................. 146

Where to Find the Science...................................... 159

About the Author.. 176

What is Happiness?

"I must learn to brook being happier than I deserve."

–JANE AUSTEN, *PERSUASION*

In an age of anxiety and uncertainty, we're all searching for ways to feel better. One in six Americans is on some kind of antidepressant. Beer, wine, and liquor sales have been on a steady incline for years ($25.2 billion in U.S. sales for 2016). Viewings of baby goat videos are up dramatically (data to come). Even those who are doing relatively well have become aware that material success does not necessarily translate into a more durable sense of well-being.

So it's no surprise that everyone is looking to add more happiness to their lives. We want to know how to stop feeling stressed and to smile more. Or how to bring more fun into our date nights. Or what kinds of plants will improve our mood (hint: Stay away from pointy leaves). With such demand to get happier, there's been perhaps an even greater supply to meet it; from feel-good inspirational quotes to in-depth scientific studies, happiness has become big business.

But the abundance of information out there can leave the average person overwhelmed. You are busy and likely just looking for some simple tips to add more fun to your day—without all the scientific jargon or unrealistic advice about the best yoga positions to save your marriage. If you're feeling stressed or unsatisfied, you're likely looking for sensible, actionable, and ultimately fun tips to help you get happy. And that's what this book aims to deliver. As you read, some of the tips might sound familiar (maybe since you're already a generally happy person) but others will, I hope, catch you by surprise or get you to see your habits or daily life in a new light.

Word of warning: I'm not a scientist or an academic, and this book is hardly a comprehensive guide to the mountain of happiness research that is out there. But it does provide some accessible insights that will help you live your life with a little more cheer and a few more laughs throughout the day. I dove into the vast amount of data available and interviewed psychologists, researchers, and happiness experts to find some of the most surprising, useful, and interesting research about happiness and how we can get more of it in our lives. *Happiness Hacks* aims to keep things light and in layperson's terms, but if you do want to dig more deeply into any of the science discussed, see the extensive endnotes with all the details on the numerous studies and researchers referenced.

But before we get started, we should probably answer the question:

What Exactly Is Happiness?

It's a question that has been pondered by everyone from Plato to Al Green, and the answers vary as widely as the people asking. The word *happiness* derives from the word for luck, as in "happenstance" or "haphazard." At least going back to before the Enlightenment, many viewed it as a matter of random luck or divine fortune if someone felt happy or not. To a degree, this is true—several researchers have made a case that happiness is genetic or hardwired into our personality. At the other end of the spectrum are those who believe happiness can be boiled down to an equation: a certain level of dopamine plus stimulation to a particular part of the brain, and *bingo*, you're happy. But for many who have looked into the question, the truth lies somewhere in the middle.

Two Types of Happiness: Instant Gratification Versus Long-Term Fulfillment

Researchers have answered the question "What is happiness?" with two different, awkward-to-pronounce adjectives: hedonic and eudaemonic. Hedonic happiness is all about maximizing pleasure and minimizing pain, and tends to be characterized as momentary or superficial. It may be the satisfaction you get from eating a great meal, or the good feeling after a workout or a successful date—whatever experience gives you, personally, enjoyment and delight.

Critics point out that using this simple "more pleasure than displeasure" equation fails to really get at what it means to be happy. These folks embrace a different definition of happiness: eudaemonic happiness, a broader sense of psychological well-being—that you are living a fulfilling life in line with your personal goals and values, and perhaps contributing to the larger good of society while you're at it. It's a concept Aristotle defined in his *Nicomachean Ethics* as a flourishing, fulfilled life, rather than a transitory feeling of pleasure, "for as it is not one swallow or one fine day that makes a spring, so it is not one day or a short time that makes a man blessed and happy."

Both forms of happiness will put a smile on your face, but each leads to a distinctly different kind of fulfillment. From a scientific perspective, assessing what can foster these different types of happiness requires different types of measurements and different criteria as well.

While the term *hedonism* is usually applied to high-living libertines looking to indulge every vice they can think of, hedonism in the study of happiness isn't just about physical pleasure. It can include your feelings about a wide range of positive and negative aspects of your life, summed up as *subjective well-being*.

Edward F. Diener, a professor of psychology at the University of Illinois at Urbana-Champaign, sees subjective well-being as the combination of three ingredients:

❶ Life satisfaction
❷ Positive mood
❸ Absence of negative mood

Put them all together, and you get your happiness level. Reflecting how happiness can be measured at different levels, Diener developed three different scales to analyze different types of happiness: the Scale of Positive and Negative Experience measures more immediate positive or negative feelings; the Satisfaction with Life Scale asks about one's general outlook on life; and the Flourishing Scale has an eight-item summary that measures one's self-perceived success in areas such as relationships and self-esteem.

Be Your True Self

But getting your immediate needs met in the form of a good meal or workout doesn't equate to true long-term happiness, according to the eudaemonic view. As developmental psychologist Alan Waterman puts it, eudaemonic happiness is "where what is considered worth desiring and having in life is the best within us or personal excellence." In other words, the marathon runner is going to achieve higher long-term happiness levels than the recreational runner who skipped out on practice to enjoy a burger.

In Waterman's study of more than 200 college students, what he calls the "personal expressiveness" of eudaemonic happiness was more strongly associated with feeling challenged, competent, and assertive, while those experiencing hedonic enjoyment were more likely to feel relaxed, content, and excited, and to have a sense of losing track of time.

So happiness is far from a simple concept. It can refer to a wide range of moods, emotions, sensations, and traits, each with its respective benefits and drawbacks.

Focus on the 40 Percent

There would not be much point to this book, or the vast happiness industry, if it were not possible to boost your happiness, at least temporarily. But researchers have found that genetic factors play a significant role in one's level of subjective well-being. For example, identical twins have been found to be much more similar in their happiness levels than fraternal twins.

Not only is happiness partly genetic, it has also been found to be a personality trait that remains stable for much of our lives. A meta-analysis covering more than 40,000 adults found that personality could, to a large degree, predict subjective well-being, life satisfaction, and happiness. "Sunny disposition" is not just an expression; people really are naturally disposed to being cheery, or melancholy, or quietly satisfied.

But while a significant part of our happiness levels is determined by things we are unlikely to change, if you feel there is not enough joy in your life, don't despair.

University of California, Riverside psychology professor and happiness expert Sonja Lyubomirsky sums this up as a pie chart in which approximately 50 percent of our happiness is genetic and 10 percent is related to life circumstances; the remaining 40 percent is under our power to change. That 40 percent can be the difference between doing pretty well and doing great, or feeling cruddy and feeling okay. And researchers have found plenty of evidence to back up the assertion that change is possible, whether through modifying work habits, taking a different approach to your communication style with friends or partners, or just rethinking the interior design of your home.

Read on for these science-based ways to positively impact that 40 percent of your happiness.

Happy at Work

"If you want to be happy, set a goal that commands your thoughts, liberates your energy, and inspires your hopes."

–ANDREW CARNEGIE

Unhappiness can be expensive. According to a Gallup-Healthways study, unhappiness is costing the United States as much as $300 billion annually in lost productivity.

Why? A higher level of life satisfaction or a cheery disposition will actually make you better at your job, more likely to get a promotion, and less likely to quit. One study of government workers found that happy people are more productive, and people are more productive when in a happy mood. Another report, out of the University of Warwick in Coventry, England, put a precise number on it: Happiness led to a 12 percent jump in productivity, while unhappy workers are 10 percent less productive than their happier peers. Sales? Thirty-seven percent higher from happy workers. Creativity? *Three times* higher.

These aren't isolated findings; a meta-analysis of 225 academic studies by some of the most prominent researchers in the field of positive psychology found direct causality between life satisfaction and positive business results.

But being happy at work is easier said than done. Even if you love your job, there's probably something you hate about it: a long commute, a boss who doesn't give you the credit you deserve, a coworker who eats lunch with their mouth open. Even if you start the day eager to dive into a project, by late afternoon you are likely struggling to stay focused. Even if you're great at what you do, there's that nagging voice in the back of your mind asking if you wouldn't be happier in another job, or if you shouldn't be getting paid more for this one.

Whatever the reason, if you're one of the majority of people who aren't exactly tap dancing to work, here are some ways to tick up your level of on-the-job happiness.

Ask: Why Are You Doing This?

It's the basic question every person should ask themself every now and then. A person is more likely to find satisfaction in their job and be better at it if they pursue work goals that are in line with their core values, or are what psychologists call "self-concordant." A pair of researchers found that those pursuing goals in line with their interests put more sustained effort into accomplishing the goals and felt a greater sense of well-being when they accomplished them.

The researchers validated this through a study of 169 students who were asked to list ten personal goals they wanted to pursue for the semester. They were asked to rank from one to ten their reasons for pursuing each goal (e.g., "you pursue this striving because of the fun and enjoyment it provides you"). Throughout the semester, they noted how much effort they were putting in toward each goal and rated their progress on each. There was a positive correlation between self-concordant goals and both effort toward and attainment of the goals, compared to those that were not. The study also found that those who achieved these goals felt a greater sense of well-being than those who pursued goals based on more external pressures.

· Ask yourself why you are working on a particular project, or even in the line of work you're pursuing. If you aren't doing it because you are passionate about it or feel it aligns with who you truly are, sooner or later, the work will become a slog.

It's Not About the Paycheck

Whatever meaning you are drawing from your job, one thing is for certain: Doing it for money won't bring you happiness. Numerous studies have found no correlation between higher salaries and higher levels of happiness. Surveys of the wealthiest Americans find their happiness scores on par with the Amish. A survey of thousands of twins found that income accounted for less than 2 percent of the difference in their respective levels of well-being.

A good rule of thumb: $80K is enough. Researchers have found that once a person earns an average of $75,000 per year, they experience a "happiness plateau." Those making millions may be able to buy nice things, but they don't enjoy a higher level of happiness commensurate with the higher salary.

When happiness does relate to a person's paycheck, it's usually in how it compares to other workers in that person's peer group. A pair of researchers drawing on data from 5,000 British workers found that their reported satisfaction levels were higher when they compared themselves to people making less than they did.

One other point they found: While absolute pay did not predict a person's sense of satisfaction, their education did—as in, the higher their education level, the lower their sense of life satisfaction. The researchers suggested that this was because of the higher aspirations that education creates.

• Stop putting so much importance on making more at work. A fatter paycheck is not going to make your smile any wider.

It's Not Even About a Really Big Paycheck

A separate study of the *Forbes* 400 richest Americans found them just slightly happier than the Maasai people of East Africa—hunter-gatherers who live in mud huts without electricity or running water.

Track Your Progress

Viewing your activities as part of a long-term goal improves your mood—on a chemical level. Participants in a study were asked about personal and family goals, rated their mood, and assessed the relevance of their current activity to these goals during the day, every three hours over a week. At each check-in, subjects also provided saliva samples so their levels of cortisol—informally known as the "stress hormone"—could be measured.

Activities that participants identified as furthering their goals correlated with more positive mood ratings and lower levels of cortisol in their saliva, suggesting that goal-oriented behavior is important to mood and stress management.

• Make a daily goal chart and track how each step forward is moving you toward accomplishing a long-term goal.

Encourage Autonomy

Researchers have found that freely choosing to take on a task maintains or even increases your energy level, while feeling controlled

SHOW YOUR HAPPINESS

Demonstrating happiness—a "positive affect," as psychologists call it—can provide a wide range of benefits. A study from the Haas School of Business at the University of California, Berkeley found that expressing positive emotions brings three distinct benefits to the workplace:

❶ It improves your own job performance (with enhanced cognitive functioning and greater persistence in working on tasks).

❷ It improves others' responses to you (with greater interpersonal attraction and making them more prone to responding favorably to your "social influence attempts," i.e., they are more likely to like you and do what you want them to do).

❸ It improves your response to others (you are more likely to help others).

In the Berkeley study, workers who displayed positive emotions at their job received more favorable supervisor evaluations and greater pay eighteen months later. The happier employees also had greater support from supervisors and coworkers.

· Smile at work, and don't be afraid to show when you're feeling happy—it can create a range of positive side effects.

tends to make your energy flag. A pair of researchers looked at samples from a pain treatment center and a weight-loss clinic. They found that those who reported more autonomy in their reasons for treatment showed more vitality, and "less vitality when they perceived themselves as controlled by external forces," as the researchers put it.

These findings can be extended to work: Even those who do not enjoy the work they are engaged in, or see it as a necessary evil, are likely to go about it with more energy if given some control or autonomy over how it's done or their reason for doing it.

· If you're a supervisor, give your staff the autonomy to choose their own tasks, or at least to schedule them at times of their choosing.

KNOW WHO YOU ARE WORKING FOR

"It's often easier to answer the why you are doing a job with who. If you care about who you work for, it's a lot easier to go the extra mile. We spoke with a pharmaceutical company that wanted to improve the motivation and job satisfaction in their company. They would show video clips of patients who used their medication and a patient might say, 'This medicine allows me to stay up one more hour to go on a date night with my husband,' or, 'This medicine allows me to play on the playground with my children.' It had a huge impact on the employees. It became very obvious to them not only why it was important, but who it was important for. They weren't producing pills, they were changing lives."

–Isabella Arendt, analyst at the Happiness Research Institute,
Copenhagen, Denmark

Ditch Contracts

While "get it in writing" is conventional wisdom in business, whether securing someone's services or buying a product, it turns out that it can actually hurt the level of trust between those involved. A pair of experiments found that binding contracts tended to inhibit levels of trust when they were in effect, since those involved tended to attribute the other person's cooperation not to their own decision, but to the "constraints imposed by the contract."

By contrast, the researchers found that nonbinding contracts did less to impede the development of interpersonal trust than binding contracts—and didn't hurt trust as much when removed. The researchers concluded that contracts not only get in the way of developing a trusting relationship in the first place, but hurt the trust between people that has already been built.

• *Unless you are striking a deal where big money is on the line, it's better for all involved to go with your gut rather than what a piece of paper requires.*

Personalize Your Space

While taking long personal calls at work to speak with your spouse or cat psychic might not be a great way to win over your boss, bringing your personal life into your workspace has been found to have very positive results. A pair of psychologists from the University of Exeter in England found that workers were more productive when their desks were "decorated rather than lean"—that is, when their desks included additions such as plants or art. In two experiments conducted by the researchers, one at a university psychology department, the other at a commercial city office, the performance of subjects (attention to detail, management of information, processing of information, and so on) was measured in four different conditions: an undecorated or "lean" workspace; one that had been decorated with plants and art by the experimenter; self-decorated; and self-decorated, then redecorated by the experimenter.

The results consistently showed that those with decorated spaces were more productive than those with lean ones. When participants had input into the decoration of their spaces, the researchers noted, it "increased participants' feelings of autonomy and decisional involvement and this led to increases in comfort, job satisfaction, and productivity." This feeling of empowerment led to an increase in productivity by as much as 32 percent.

· *Add some artwork or plants to your desk, or make some other addition that enhances it in a way that's personal for you. Throw in a lava lamp and disco ball if you're into that sort of thing.*

Get Plants

In a separate study by the same lead researchers, they compared lean to "green" workspaces. In a trio of experiments, workers in places where plants had been added reported higher levels of job satisfaction, concentration, and perceived air quality. The researchers concluded that workers who put household plants on their desks were 15 percent more productive than those who did not. An eighteen-month study on this phenomenon published in the *Journal of Experimental Psychology: Applied* found that call center workers who had plants on their desks had better memory retention and performed better at their tasks.

Walk to Work, or Get a Bike

When it comes to commutes, it may not be the length that matters. While some research has found that longer commutes tend to correlate with lower job satisfaction, a study of 3,400 people by scientists at McGill University in Montreal examined six different modes of transportation for getting to work and respondents' relative satisfaction. Subjects were interviewed in both the summer and winter to get an average satisfaction score that accounted for changing weather conditions (biking in a blizzard isn't satisfactory, you'd assume). They found that while the commute length did not correlate with satisfaction, the mode of transportation did. Specifically, the study returned the following percentages of satisfaction:

- Walkers: 85 percent
- Rail travelers: 84 percent
- Cyclists: 82 percent
- Drivers: 77 percent
- Metro/subway riders: 76 percent
- Bus riders: 75.5 percent

REVISIT WHY YOU TOOK THE JOB

"If you aren't satisfied with your job, ask yourself, 'Why did you take this job in the first place?' Somewhere down the line you applied for this job and convinced someone to pay you to do it. Either you are really good at lying to yourself, or you were motivated to do this at the time. You may realize the job has changed: now you work with a completely different customer or a product you don't really support or a different division. You may be able to reignite your motivation for the job again, or it may be time to find another job."

–Isabella Arendt

Write Down Meaningful Moments

Researcher and happiness expert Shawn Achor found that when workers spent two minutes to take four quick actions, it improved their happiness over the long term. Those four actions are:

1. Write down a meaningful experience you had in the past twenty-four hours.
2. Jot down three things you are grateful for.
3. Write a positive message to someone on Facebook or another social media site.
4. Meditate.

Participants took a well-being survey before commencing the experiment, scoring an average of 22.96 on a 35-point scale. After three weeks of doing these actions every day, this score rose to 27.23.

A separate Harvard study found that workers who made daily notes of their successes from the day in a journal enjoyed a higher level of creativity and motivation.

* *Pick up a journal and jot down your successes and meaningful experiences, and express gratitude.*

Focus on Strengths

Some people are detail oriented; others are much better at the big picture. Some are great collaborating with groups; others thrive in isolation. A manager who wants to get the most out of her team will learn to recognize the strengths of her workers. Research from Gallup backs up the value of doing work or filling roles based on personal strengths and natural talents. In a survey of just over 1,000 US employees, the organization found a strong connection between

CRAFT YOUR JOB

Don't just do your job; craft it. That's the insight from a team of researchers who urge employees to reframe their worklife in terms of their own personal strengths and passions. Called "job crafting," the exercise directs a person to "visualize the job, map its elements, and reorganize them to better suit you." Drawing on their research with companies of a wide range of sizes, they found that workers who practice this exercise grow more engaged in their work and deliver a stronger performance.

Job crafting involves a series of steps:

❶ Create a "before diagram" of what your job consists of, with larger squares representing tasks that require the most time, and smaller squares for those jobs that take less time.

❷ Review the diagram and identify areas of greatest importance—such as professional development or revenue-generating tasks—where more time should be applied.

❸ Identify your own motives, strengths, and passions—the things that inspire you to work hard or get you excited about your work.

❹ Use these to create an "after diagram" with a new set of task blocks that align with these drives, and frame your roles in a way most meaningful to you.

those who felt their supervisor focused on their strengths and active engagement in their work. By contrast, of the one quarter of workers who felt their supervisor ignored their strengths, 40 percent were actively disengaged. Interestingly, when supervisors focused on workers' weaknesses, their disengagement was just 22 percent. Apparently, even negative attention is better than no attention at all.

· *Try to figure out your employees' biggest strengths—sometimes even they don't know what those are—and ensure that they are doing work that taps into those talents.*

CUT DOWN ROLES

"When people have many different self-identities, they don't seem to fare as well at work. When you have too many roles you can get stretched too thin and it's hard to master them all. Whether self-esteem or depression or stress-related illnesses, when people have many different self-identities they tend to suffer because they are juggling too much and not sticking the landing on any of them. The main thing is to say 'no' and pare down."

–Allen McConnell, University Distinguished Professor, Department of Psychology, Miami University (Oxford, OH)

Take a Proper Break

Long live the coffee break! Researchers at the University of Toronto found that frequent breaks improve creativity. John Trougakos, associate professor of organizational behavior and HR management who coauthored the study, pointed out that our brains have a limited amount of energy, requiring them to be frequently recharged. But the researchers emphasized that just taking a break is not the solution—it's what you do with it. Specifically, to recover from work, you need to use your break to do activities that "stop the demands associated with work." That means engaging in what they defined as "respite activities"—involving either low effort (napping, relaxing, or sitting quietly) or a preferred choice (reading a book, spending time with friends). But they distinguished these respites from "chores" like running errands or tidying a desk, which don't allow you to fully recharge.

· *Avoid filling your breaks with more work (even if it's different from the work you are paid to do). Use your respite to fully recover and get your energy back for when you return to the desk.*

. . . For 17 Minutes Off, 52 Minutes On

Time-tracking productivity app DeskTime isolated the top 10 percent of the most productive employees, analyzing their computer use over a workday. Those who did the most productive work took an average break of 17 minutes, and worked straight through for 52 minutes.

. . . Or for 5 Minutes Off, 25 Minutes On

An alternate strategy is the Pomodoro Technique, in which one breaks up the workday into 30-minute sections, working for 25 minutes (1 Pomodoro, so named because the technique's inventor timed these sections on his tomato-shaped timer) at a time and breaking for 5.

Don't Eat Lunch at Your Desk

Put down that sad desk salad! However long your break runs, the key is to make it a true break, getting out of the office and fully relaxing during the time off. So stay away from business lunches when at all possible.

Don't Become a Lawyer

Maybe it's all those lawyer jokes, but those who practice law have been found to be particularly unhappy. Researchers point to three main causes of lawyer unhappiness. First, prudence is one of the main qualifications for lawyers, which can often translate into skepticism or pessimism. Second, the high pressure put on and low influence given to young associates are the sort of work conditions that result in low morale in other workplaces. Third, the work—at least in the United States—is often a zero-sum game where your win is someone else's loss, creating a hypercompetitiveness that also drains one's sense of workplace satisfaction.

A study by Johns Hopkins University found that lawyers were 3.6 times more likely than nonlawyers to suffer from depression, and other research connected the legal profession to higher levels of substance abuse.

. . . Unless You Take a Pay Cut

An exception: Lawyers in public service jobs. Public defenders, legal aid attorneys, and others in similarly low-paying but personally rewarding lines of work were most likely to report feeling happy in a survey of 6,200 lawyers. No correlation between happiness and high income or prestigious positions was found, and junior partners reported identical levels of well-being as senior associates who made 62 percent more than them.

WHAT ARE THE HAPPIEST JOBS?

CareerBliss analyzed tens of thousands of employees' self-reports about their satisfaction on the job, evaluating a huge list of different job titles, and determined these were the ten happiest of 2017:

1. Marketing specialist
2. Recruiter
3. Graduate teaching assistant
4. .NET developer
5. Director of marketing
6. Directional driller
7. QA analyst
8. Technical lead
9. Senior engineer
10. Network administrator

WHAT ARE THE UNHAPPIEST JOBS?

The same report determined these were the least happy jobs one could have:

1. Customer service representative
2. Retail cashier
3. Retail salesperson
4. Registered nurse
5. Sales account manager
6. General manager
7. Field service engineer
8. Data analyst
9. Project engineer
10. Administrative assistant

"Teams that listen to each other are happier. Leaders can model good listening and keep interruptions to a minimum during discussions. Doing these small things creates a more inclusive culture that engenders a sense of being respected and belonging."

–Kathryn Stanley, chair, Organizational and Leadership Psychology Department, William James College (Newton, MA)

Working Less Won't Make You Happier

You've probably thought now and then that maybe the root of your frustration with work is that you are working too many hours. The Happiness Research Institute, based in Denmark, looked into this claim and found mixed results, at best. In its annual survey of almost 8,000 Danes, the organization found lower job satisfaction levels among those who worked fewer hours. The researchers suggested this may be due to the fact that the respondents actually want to work more hours, or that they work fewer hours because there is less to do and their job is less stimulating than something more demanding of their time.

Several studies of working people found that those who are employed for a full forty hours a week feel higher levels of satisfaction in their lives than those who work part-time. A reduction in hours is generally accompanied by a drop in happiness, while a shift from part-time to full-time employment increases happiness (though if you're already working full-time, taking on an eighty-hour week will almost certainly *not* double your level of happiness). Even those out of work will find a greater sense of happiness by putting a full day's work into finding a new job.

· *If you find your workweek is dragging, it's probably the job, rather than the schedule, that needs to change.*

Don't Retire Early

Retiring early may be the dream for many: Who wouldn't want to cut out the nine-to-five existence by the age of fifty—or thirty? But before withdrawing from the working world to spend your days sipping piña coladas, consider that early retirement might not be great for your mind or happiness. Cross-sectional studies find workers who retire early to be less happy than those who stay in the workforce through age sixty-five.

Additional studies find a connection between retirement and memory—what a pair of economists call "mental retirement." Drawing on memory-test data from the United States, England, and eleven European countries, they found that the earlier people retired, the more their cognitive abilities declined.

Though the research does not indicate the specific elements of work that might help maintain one's mental sharpness, the study's coauthor, Robert J. Willis, told *The New York Times* that even if the work itself is not stimulating, "There is evidence that social skills and personality skills—getting up in the morning, dealing with people, knowing the value of being prompt and trustworthy—are also important."

Meditate

One of the most consistent findings of positive psychologists has been the benefits of meditation on one's ability to focus and produce good work. Researchers at Johns Hopkins University found that meditation can quiet fear and anxiety throughout the day. A study at Leiden University in the Netherlands showed that subjects who practiced "open-monitoring meditation" came up with a wider range of ideas and put themselves in a more creative state of mind.

• *Set aside a few minutes each day to meditate. While researchers suggest a twenty-minute meditation session is ideal, even just taking five minutes to stop and focus on breathing has been found to make a significant impact on your ability to work.*

Take Up Yoga

Alternatively, if your job is stressing you out, break out that downward-facing dog. A study of workers in the UK found that those who practiced weekly fifty-minute sessions of yoga for eight weeks reported lower stress levels and less back pain than those who did not do yoga.

Happy at Play

"Happiness is thought to depend on leisure; for we are busy that we may have leisure, and make war that we may live in peace."

–ARISTOTLE

When we hear "leisure," we think "fun." But not all free time makes people equally happy. Some activities are a blast in the moment but can make you feel like crap the next day (e.g., the things you did for fun in college). Others may nourish your life satisfaction for years but not feel all that fun while you're doing them. Sometimes finding happiness in your free time is all about getting out of your comfort zone; other times it's about rolling into your favorite bar with the same people you see almost every day.

So how should you be spending your time to maximize your happiness?

This question is more important than ever as leisure has become a central part of our daily lives. In a comparison of attitudes in 1938 and 2014, the role of leisure as a way to bring happiness to one's life rose from eighth place to third place (first and second in 2014 were "economic stability" and "good sense of humor," respectively). We have more free time than we ever had in decades past, but we have more mindless distractions to fill it, so we must choose how to spend our time—and how much of it we spend doing each activity—wisely.

Here are some science-backed ways to do just that.

Choose Happiness-Boosting Activities

Some activities have more impact than others on improving your happiness. That was among the findings in a survey of leisure activities in thirty-three countries and how they affected peoples' well-being. Of the thirteen different ways to pass the time that were examined, only six were found to be significantly associated with feelings of happiness:

- Shopping
- Reading books
- Attending cultural events
- Getting together with relatives
- Listening to music
- Attending sporting events

Six other activities were found to have no impact on happiness levels: watching TV, going to the movies, getting together with friends, playing cards, going to the gym, and doing handicrafts. Just one activity—spending time on the internet—was found to be negatively associated with happiness.

Make Contacts

Leisure activities can often be ends in themselves. But while having fun does have plenty of benefits, longer-term happiness comes from other aspects of leisure activities than how long they last. The same survey of thirty-three countries found that there was a higher degree of happiness gained from activities in which participants felt they established "useful contacts" and were able to "develop important skills." The takeaway? Seek out leisure activities that will give you more than just fun—those that will allow you to advance as a person and fulfill larger goals in life.

· Join the company softball team, or take up a hobby where you're likely to meet others in your career field.

Get Outside

One of the best happiness-enhancing leisure activities is to get into nature. Researchers have found that people who have spent two weeks in the wilderness enjoy a higher level of attention, a greater level of life satisfaction, and a more positive outlook after they return. On top of that, people who have spent time in the wilderness report a sense of belonging to something greater than themselves, and renewed clarity on "what really matters."

Biologist E. O. Wilson developed a "biophilia hypothesis" that suggests that humans have evolved a need to affiliate with the natural world; this explains why this "nature connectedness" might help foster a greater sense of well-being.

· Go camping for a weekend, or go for a long hike. Immerse yourself in the natural world. For a faster fix, add a ten-minute walk to your daily routine.

Head to the Park

Greenery doesn't have to be out in the wilderness to reduce your stress and increase your happiness. Evidence shows that even a relatively small amount of vegetation—small parks and urban green spaces close to one's home—can make a significant impact on well-being. Researchers in Finland found that those who spent as little as twenty minutes walking through a park felt much more relief of their stress levels than those who spent twenty minutes wandering through the center of the city.

Going to a park can also strengthen social connections since, as a researcher reviewing the literature on the subject notes, "natural elements, especially trees, encourage people to spend more time outside, making them more likely to have the accidental face-to-face encounters with their neighbors that create friendships and other social ties."

· *Go for a twenty-minute walk in the park. It will lower your stress level and you might meet someone while you're there.*

CONNECT WITH NATURE

"People who describe themselves as more connected to nature, who see themselves as a part of nature, also report more happiness—more positive emotions and purpose in life. . . . It's not that people who live in rural areas, who are surrounded by nature, are off-the-charts happy compared to people in cities. In cities, the people who find themselves near parks where there are some trees, these are the people who are happier. The little things matter: parks, gardens, even bird feeders."

–John M. Zelenski, professor of psychology, Carleton University
(Ottawa, Ontario)

. . . Or Sit by a Window

Even just looking at nature can improve your mood. In a classic study at Texas A&M University, 120 subjects were shown a stressful video, then shown a video of one of six natural or urban settings. Those who watched the natural settings showed faster and more complete recovery from stress, as measured in biometrics such as blood pressure and muscle tension.

Join a Sport

Physical activity is great for your health, of course, helping to reduce obesity and boost your physical wellness. But researchers drawing on national survey data of individuals as well as data on access to sports and fitness facilities have also found that participating in physical activity leads to a higher reported quality of life.

The researchers found that regardless of participants' personal background, those who were more actively involved in sports and physical activity reported higher levels of life satisfaction in general. In fact, participating in physical activity was found to increase happiness at three times the level that one's feeling of happiness *decreases* upon becoming unemployed.

Not only do sports association members report being happier than nonsporty people—they also report being happier than those who participate in recreation activities found outside of the realm of sports. Beyond increased health, the happiness value of sports is found in the intimate social relationships formed between players, coaches, and even opponents.

· *Sign up for a sports team—any team: baseball, badminton, hop-scotch, whatever.*

Make Leisure a Habit

Joining a sports team has another advantage: It creates a long-term habit of physical activity. A study compared the benefits of "routine" leisure activities (such as regular meet-ups with friends, or team sports) versus "project-based" ones (such as a volunteer project or one-time competitions). Drawing on responses from 365 college students, the researchers found that *routine* leisure brings happiness and meaning to life.

• *Make consistent physical leisure-time activity part of your life, as opposed to just doing one-off outings. Find some way to make fun activities something you will continue for months or years.*

Value Time over Money

Money can't buy love—or happiness, it turns out. Researchers at the University of Pennsylvania and the University of California, Los Angeles used online surveys to poll more than 4,000 people on the question of whether they would rather have more time or more money—and whether they were happy. While 64 percent of respondents said they would prefer to have more money, it was those who preferred more time who reported being the happiest.

Though the researchers acknowledged this may be the case because those with plenty of money may be happier—and also prefer more time since they don't need the money—they emphasized that "what matters is the value people place on each resource and not necessarily the amount of time or money they have (or feel they have)."

• *Stop for a moment and appreciate the moments you have.*

Buy Experiences, Not Things

Along the same lines, this money/time dichotomy correlates to the relationship that researchers have consistently found between *things* and *experiences*. You've heard it before: Paying for experiences (vacations, spa treatments, even trips to the movies) has been found to create more long-term pleasure than buying material goods. But this truth pops up again and again in a number of different ways. In a survey by Harvard University psychology professor Dan Gilbert, 57 percent of respondents reported greater happiness from experiential purchases compared with 34 percent who gained more happiness from material objects.

Beyond that, the emotional benefits you get from buying an experience are likely to exceed your expectations. In a different study, Ryan Howell of San Francisco State University asked participants to rate on a scale from one to seven whether they felt their money would be well spent on different types of purchases. Respondents expected material purchases would bring them an average satisfaction score of 4.41, while experiential purchases only earned a 2.9 rating. Two weeks after making the buy, the higher number flipped: respondents gave material purchases a 4.91 average, and experiential purchases a 5.7 average rating.

To top it off, researchers from Cornell University and the University of Colorado Boulder found in a pair of surveys and a follow-up laboratory experiment that people get more pleasure in *anticipating* experiences than they do looking forward to making a material purchase. The researchers determined this was the case because experiences are more open to positive reinterpretations, are more closely related to a person's identity, and contribute more to social relationships (you're going to tell people about your upcoming vacation more than your upcoming furniture purchase). So before, during, and after purchase, experiences beat things.

· Instead of buying a new pair of shoes, spend that money on a staycation.

Take Eight-Day Vacations

Speaking of vacations, one of the worst feelings in the world is having taken off a few days from work, only to come back feeling like the relaxation didn't really stick. It may be that the vacation you took wasn't long enough—or it may have been *too* long. A group of workers answered a questionnaire about health and well-being prior to and during vacations that averaged 23 days each (yes, these were European workers). Researchers found that feelings of health and well-being increased right away during vacation, then peaked on the eighth day, where they remained until the eleventh day, after which enjoyment levels faded out. From this, the researchers suggest that eight days is about how long it takes to let go of concerns about work responsibilities and stress—but before feelings of homesickness or restlessness set in.

· Tack your next one-week vacation onto a three-day weekend to stretch it to a little more than a week—but just a little.

Plan Vacations Earlier

Sadly, no matter how long a vacation may be, its impact *after* you return to work is likely to be minimal. The same study found that on the first day of work resumption, the positive health and well-being effects from the time off vanished entirely.

Before you despair that a break will never truly refresh you, the secret might be to put greater weight on what happens *before* the vacation itself. Beyond actually going on an extended holiday, simply planning or thinking about taking a trip can boost your overall happiness. That was the finding of a team of researchers in the Netherlands who surveyed 1,530 Dutch adults about their feelings of happiness before and after taking a vacation. While they similarly found that feelings of happiness and relaxation dropped off after a trip, they discovered that the largest boost in happiness came in the planning stages of a getaway. Vacationers displayed higher levels of happiness than nonvacationers for weeks, and sometimes even months, before the holiday began.

• *Start planning your next trip months in advance. You'll give yourself plenty of time to imagine lying on the beach, wandering historic city streets, or whatever else your ideal escape involves (plus save money on the flight).*

Have Fun First

Sometimes it may be better to have your dessert before dinner. We often think that we will enjoy a leisure activity or vacation as a reward for getting our work done, but it turns out we'll have just as much fun playing *before* working. Researchers at the University of Chicago Booth School of Business tapped 181 adults from a wide range of employment backgrounds to complete two activities: a set of cognitive tests (aka work) and an iPad game in which participants created and listened to music (aka play). While participants expected that having fun first would decrease their enjoyment of playing the game, in fact there turned out to be no difference between the two.

The researchers got the same results with an experiment in which 259 college students had a choice to enjoy a spa treatment either before their midterms or as a destressing experience after taking their tests. Again, the enjoyment was the same whether before or after. Ed O'Brien, coauthor of the study, said the findings "suggest we may be over-worrying and over-working for future rewards that could be just as pleasurable in the present."

· *Stop postponing play. Take that vacation or go out for the day, even if you haven't finished that project you've been stressing about.*

DON'T EXPECT BALANCE *EVERY* DAY

"Most people think of 'work/life balance' as reflecting an ability to balance work and home life on a daily basis, by, for example, working an adequate amount of time but then having enough time each day to unwind, relax, and engage in enjoyable leisure activities. That's great, but sometimes unachievable. For example, I'm currently working on a book and for the last seven months or so, pretty much if I'm awake, I'm working. There's no balance. But, I do expect to slow down and find some recovery time once the book is done. Sometimes you can achieve balance every day or every week, and sometimes balance gets put on the back shelf and waits until the time is right."

–Jamie Gruman, associate professor of organizational behavior, University of Guelph (Guelph, Ontario)

You're More Competent on the Weekend

Just as breaks during the day are found to correlate with higher levels of happiness and productivity, weekends are key to helping raise your level of happiness. Research finds a "weekend effect" among workers in every field, in which their mood improves from Friday afternoon to Sunday evening.

A study tracked the moods of participants over a three-week period and consistently found that respondents reported feeling both mentally and physically better on the weekend, regardless of age, marital status, or other factors. The subjects also reported feeling more competent on the weekend than during the week, likely because they had more freedom to choose the activities they wanted to do. "Far from frivolous, the relatively unfettered time on weekends provides critical opportunities for bonding with others, exploring interests and relaxing—basic psychological needs that people should be careful not to crowd out with overwork," said Richard Ryan, a psychology professor at the University of Rochester, who authored the study.

Go with the Flow

One good litmus test for whether your leisure activities will bring you happiness is to ask yourself, "Does it put me in a flow state?" Positive psychologist Mihály Csíkszentmihályi coined the term *flow* to describe the kind of hyperfocus that he defines as "being completely involved in an activity for its own sake. The ego falls away. Time flies." You know what he's talking about: Maybe you were totally engrossed in a great book or rode your bike all afternoon and lost track of the day. You were "in the zone" and went on a kind of euphoric autopilot. In this flow state, you can accomplish more creative work and do so much more effectively or creatively than in your typical distracted state—all while being more relaxed and positive.

Csíkszentmihályi laid out the factors that contribute to a sense of flow, including intense focus and concentration, a feeling of personal control over what you are working on, a distorted experience of time (i.e., time flies), and a loss of the sense of self-consciousness. To enter the flow state, the key is engaging in a task that balances with your skills. Something too simple leads to boredom; something too challenging leads to anxiety. While the flow state can happen in any area of life, sports and outdoor activities are often where it can be seen at its clearest.

• *Aim to reach flow state when having fun: Seek out activities that challenge your skills but won't overwhelm you, and cut out distractions while you're having fun.*

Flow in Teams

Getting into flow is not something that has to be done solo. A research team from St. Bonaventure University in upstate New York asked subjects to participate in a paddleball activity, both by themselves and with a team, meant to trigger a sense of flow individually and as part of a group. It turned out that students got greater satisfaction from "social flow" than from "solitary flow."

• *Turn your hobbies into group activities: If you like playing guitar, start a band; if you love jogging, run races.*

Find an Adventure

Adventure outings have been found to be particularly effective at creating this sense of flow—even when generating feelings of anxiety at the same time. One study surveyed fifty-two white-water kayakers, analyzing their experiences with kayaking and subsequent feelings. It found that even when subjects expressed feeling anxious due to the difficulty of the river, these emotions were counterbalanced by subjective experiences of flow, "suggesting that white-water kayakers may have positive experiences even when their abilities are exceeded by the difficulty of the river," as the researchers put it. They also found that those who experienced a flow state continued to feel its effects even after the more difficult parts of the rapids had passed, making it seem that "benefits from the flow experience may be taken away from the river into everyday life."

• *Challenge yourself with an adventurous outing. The butterflies you feel can create long-term mood improvement.*

Knit . . . or Quilt

But you don't have to put yourself in harm's way to improve your sense of happiness. It turns out that knitting is an effective way to boost your mood. A survey of 3,545 knitters found a notable connection between how frequently someone knitted and their feelings of calm and happiness. Those who knitted more frequently also reported sharper concentration and memory.

Part of that might be yarn itself: Some respondents reported that the color they used while knitting influenced their mood. About half of respondents said the texture—what some referred to as "tactile pleasures in fibers" and "touchable feelable result"—impacted their mood.

Similar findings came from a survey of quilters. Those taking part in a survey about quilting and well-being reported higher levels of concentration and emotional benefits, thanks to the strong social network generated from interacting with others in a quilting circle.

• *Visit a craft store and start a new hobby—with friends, if possible.*

Get Playful

Playfulness—reframing a situation to be more amusing or fun—is something we have an instinct for as children (who hasn't turned couch cushions into an impenetrable fort or a jungle gym into a castle?), even if as adults we can lose our appreciation of play. But it turns out that reactivating it is a great way to bolster happiness.

In a study of 255 adults, subjects rated their playfulness (using the five-question Short Measure of Adult Playfulness survey, as well as the thirty-two-adjective Adult Playfulness Scale) and their life satisfaction, and stated how often they engaged in activities they enjoyed. The researchers found a correlation between playfulness and both high levels of life satisfaction and an inclination to take part in enjoyable activities and to live an active lifestyle.

· *Turn something boring into a game: Give a goofy name when your barista asks, or imagine your commute as a high-stakes obstacle course.*

DROP THE "NOT ENOUGH TIME" EXCUSE

"Most people in our research over the years give the major reason for not participating in leisure activities as 'not enough time.' However, we should distrust this explanation and more often than not treat it as an 'excuse.' In our time-use studies, we have found that when people say they don't have enough time to engage in physically active leisure or other more demanding and potentially satisfying activities, for example, they are watching three to four hours of television a day. Time constraints do not really seem to be the issue, rather it's a question of priorities."

–Roger C. Mannell, Distinguished Professor Emeritus and former dean, Faculty of Applied Health Sciences, University of Waterloo (Waterloo, Ontario)

Crack a Joke

Just like playfulness, laughter really can be powerful medicine. Paul McGhee, who has spent two decades researching humor and laughter, has found lots of evidence that humor boosts emotional resilience and helps people cope with stress, even reducing pain and strengthening people's immune systems. Even better—he's found that a sense of humor is something that can be learned and improved with practice. McGhee lays out a program of "7 Humor Habits" that have been found to strengthen a person's funny muscles, including "surround yourself with humor," "laugh more often and more heartily," and "laugh at yourself." He maintains that adding humor to one's life creates a cognitive shift in perspective and provides individuals with a greater sense of control and feeling of empowerment.

Researchers at the James Cook University in Cairns, Australia, sought to test these assertions, randomly assigning fifty-five participants to three groups: one that followed McGhee's eight-week humor skills program (complete with a handbook of jokes and funny stories), one that met weekly for social gatherings, and a control group. Far more than the other two groups, those who went through the program of learning to laugh more and find humor in difficult situations showed a significant increase in positive affect, optimism, and perception of control over their surroundings. They also reported decreases in perceived stress, depression, and anxiety levels.

• *Take an improv class or pick up a joke book. You don't have to be a natural class clown to improve your sense of humor.*

. . . But Not at Someone Else's Expense

One of the most attractive traits anyone can have is a sense of humor, but some types of funny are less healthy than others. Researchers asked forty-three males and sixty-six females to complete questionnaires about their humor styles, subjective happiness, and affective styles. The results indicated that practicing aggressive or "self-defeating" humor used to belittle or tease correlated with lower levels of happiness, while positive or "self-enhancing" humor led to higher happiness levels. "Self-directed humor" also had a stronger correlation with happiness ratings than did humor directed toward others.

· *Skip the sarcastic, aggressive, negative humor focusing on other people's weaknesses.*

Limit Your Options

Being able to choose what to do or what to buy is usually a good thing. But too many choices can be a bummer. Anyone who has felt overwhelmed trying to decide how to spend a day off or what to order from one of those thirty-page diner menus can appreciate that having a lot of options can sometimes feel the opposite of liberating. There is such a thing as too much of a good thing.

Researchers at Stanford and Columbia Universities looked into why this might be the case by offering one group of subjects thirty different types of chocolates from which they could choose a sample, and another group just six types of chocolate. The subjects then answered a few questions about how much satisfaction they felt about their selection. Those choosing from the larger variety reported more regret and dissatisfaction with their final decision. When given the option, they said they were less likely to choose chocolates instead of money as compensation for participating in the study, while those with fewer to choose from were more eager for more chocolate.

The researchers suggest that "[p]erhaps it is not that people are made unhappy by the decisions they make in the face of abundant options, but that they are instead unsure—that they are burdened by the responsibility of distinguishing good from bad decisions."

· *Use a bracket approach when making a decision between many options, cutting down each choice to a selection between two things: Do you like A or B more? If you like A more, how does it stack up to C? And so on.*

Become a Bar Regular

Speaking of finding happiness in limited options, you don't have to travel to far-flung places to boost your well-being. *Happy hour* at your favorite bar might be a more accurate term than you realized. A team of Oxford psychologists and anthropologists in England found that people who have a "local" that they frequent had more close friends on whom they could count for support, and were found to be happier with their lives, more embedded in their communities, and more trusting of others. These conclusions drew on a poll from UK-based data analytics firm YouGov of 2,254 UK adults, in which the 22 percent of respondents who said they had a favorite pub had an average of 7.2 close friends, compared with the average of 6.0 friends for those who did not have a favorite bar.

Lead researcher Robin Dunbar chalked it up to the personal connections created at the local watering hole, stating that making and maintaining friendships is "done face-to-face: the digital world is simply no substitute."

· *Find your own Cheers in your neighborhood and get to know everybody's name.*

Listen with Intention

Positive music can help you feel happier—if you want it to. A pair of psychology professors looked at how music affects happiness levels. They asked a group of subjects to listen to twelve minutes of music, including the "positive" (i.e., upbeat) *Rodeo* by Aaron Copland and the less-cheery *Rite of Spring* by Igor Stravinsky, noting how the music impacted their moods. The more positive music did indeed boost the subjects' happiness levels—but only when listeners put "intention" behind their listening.

Over the two-week period the test was conducted, those who listened to the positive music after being asked to try to feel happier reported a more positive mood. Those participants who listened to Stravinsky's piece, regardless of instructions, and those who listened to Copland without being told to think happy thoughts, had no significant change of mood. The researchers concluded that the combination of the right music *and* the right thoughts is important in increasing positive feelings. One without the other is not enough.

· *Listen to upbeat music to increase your happiness level—but pause to think positive thoughts before pressing play.*

Cool Down

Sunshine on your face feels great, but a researcher at Osaka University in Japan has found that happiness is likely to be maxed out at a slightly cool temperature, specifically 57 degrees Fahrenheit (13.9 degrees Celsius). Examining the effect of weather on well-being, the researcher gathered data on seventy-five students over a period of 516 days, controlling for individual characteristics and outside events. He found that while wind speed and precipitation did not impact respondents' well-being, subjective happiness was negatively related to temperature and humidity, with subjects at their happiest at 57 degrees Fahrenheit.

· *If you're feeling down, turn up the air conditioner.*

Do Something for Someone Else

Enough about you. Instead of doing things for your own happiness, you should set aside some time each month to do something that helps someone else. Why? It will make you happier. Tons of psychological studies have found evidence of the paradoxical relationship between selflessness and happiness—that is, by giving to others and avoiding selfish behavior, you end up gaining in the process.

In a series of studies, researchers found that "prosocial behavior" (actions focused on others, such as giving money to those in need) boosted a person's feelings of happiness upon recalling it later. Researchers conducted three experiments to test this. One involved getting eighty-six participants to recall a memory of their choice that involved spending twenty dollars, either on themselves or for someone else. After recalling the memory, they completed a survey on how they felt—and those who recalled spending for others reported more positive emotions.

* *Designate two hours each month to serve at a soup kitchen or do some other kind of volunteer work. You'll end up feeling better as a result—but remember: It's not about you.*

HƏPPY iN LOVe

*"Happiness quite unshared can scarcely be
called happiness—it has no taste."*

–CHARLOTTE BRONTË

When it comes to boosting your happiness, few areas are as important as your love life. George Vaillant, a researcher behind the milestone Harvard Grant Study (which followed 268 Harvard undergraduates for more than seventy-five years), states that "[h]appiness is love. Full stop." Everything from life expectancy to confidence to stress levels is impacted by your romantic relationships, and your decisions and personality in turn shape the success of your love life.

Almost nothing in life is as mysterious and deeply personal as love. So it can seem reductive to turn a complex relationship into cold data points, unnatural to put a number on something so personal as how many times a husband compliments his wife, or how many times a couple has sex in a month. But just as Shakespeare, Neruda, and Keats have sought to understand what makes for ideal love, in more recent times psychologists and researchers have made their own attempts at solving the puzzle. The results have been less poetic, but no less insightful.

From the importance of a great "how we met story" to the best time to break things off, researchers have explored virtually every aspect of what makes a relationship work—and what doesn't. Here are some takeaways from their findings on how to create a more successful love life and, as a result, a happier life.

Five Is the Magic Number

Whether a couple stays together or not may come down to a simple equation. Famed relationship psychologist John Gottman found through reviewing two decades of observational research that marriages that last maintain a ratio of positive-to-negative interactions of about five to one. The researcher found a mean positivity ratio of 5.1 to 1 for "speech acts" and 4.7 to 1 for "observed emotions."

Those who exhibit closer to a one-to-one ratio of positive to negative are likely to "cascade to divorce," according to the researcher. In 1992, Gottman and a pair of mathematicians recruited 700 newly married couples, videotaping fifteen-minute conversations between the two and counted the number of positive and negative interactions. They were able to predict whether the couples would still be together a decade later with 94 percent accuracy.

· *Track your interactions with your partner over the course of a day. How frequently are you complimenting or expressing affection? How often are you criticizing or expressing frustration? If the ratio of positive-to-negative expressions is less than five to one, work to move that needle.*

Wait at Least a Month for Sex

Whatever your policy on one-night stands, if you're looking to build a long-term relationship, odds are better if you don't rush into things.

Relationship researchers have noted for years that couples who cohabit before engagement and marriage are more likely to divorce—in part because they are more likely to shift into marriage more through inertia than an active choice. But it turns out that hopping into bed immediately does not bode well for a relationship, either.

Cornell University researcher Sharon Sassler conducted a study of almost 600 married and cohabiting couples, surveying them about their relationship quality, sexual satisfaction, and communication. Controlling for variables such as age, income, and number of children, the researchers found that those who had sex within a month of starting to date (more than one third of respondents) reported lower relationship satisfaction. For the women surveyed, the longer they waited for sex, the better their perception of their current relationship.

· *If you see longer-term potential in the person you just started dating, hold off on sex—at least for a few weeks.*

Do a Daily Debrief

Communication is key to successful relationships, but often communication takes the form of discussing what you're going to eat for dinner or figuring out who has to walk the dog. Drawing on her longitudinal study of 373 couples over decades, psychologist Terri Orbuch found that 98 percent of happy couples agreed that they "intimately know and understand" their partner. Additionally, a majority of happy spouses said they "often" revealed intimate things to their spouses, while just 19 percent of unhappy couples did the same.

To that end, she recommends that couples practice the Ten-Minute Rule, in which every day the couple discusses for ten minutes any topic *except* household responsibilities, work, or kids. From Orbuch's findings, the daily habit of chatting about nonwork

REPAIR YOUR RELATIONSHIP HOUSE

Just as the home you live in is (hopefully) built carefully with sturdy materials, so too should your relationship be. John Gottman and his fellow psychologist (and wife) Julie Gottman developed a mathematical system—or what might be better described as an architectural system—for whether a couple would remain together or divorce, based on physiological data collected while the pair of subjects got into a disagreement. The Gottman's used decades of their research to create the "sound relationship house theory," which outlines seven levels of a successful love relationship.

❶ Build love maps: Get to know the inner workings of your partner by asking open-ended questions.

❷ Share fondness and admiration: Focus on the good things about your partner, creating a habit of appreciation.

❸ Turn toward instead of away: Answer your partner's bids for attention and support (see next page).

❹ Positive perspective: View your partner through rose-colored glasses, giving them the benefit of the doubt and avoiding what's called "negative sentiment override"– defaulting to a negative view of your partner.

❺ Manage conflict: Identify negative patterns in the relationship and either resolve them when possible, or create an ongoing dialogue with your partner about the problem.

❻ Achieve life dreams: Help your partner to accomplish their long-term goals and life dreams.

❼ Create shared meaning, the "attic" of the house: Share experiences, stories, and visions of the relationship's future.

subjects opens the door to personal topics that will help you better know your spouse in a more intimate way.

Seek Out "Bids"

The third level of the Gottmans' relationship house (see previous page) is "turn toward instead of away," based on studying newlyweds and following up with them six years later. The couples who remained married had something in common: When one member of the couple made a "bid"—for attention, affection, or some other kind of connection—the other member of the couple acknowledged it and responded positively. As an example: If your partner asks, "How do I look?," she is both asking a question and bidding for your attention and you should give her a positive response ("You look amazing!"). Or it may be a nonverbal bid, like putting her head on your shoulder, in which case you should affirm your partner nonverbally in response, such as by wrapping your arm around her.

In the Gottmans' research, members of the couples who stayed married over the six years responded to these bids an average of 86 percent of the time. Those who divorced responded only 33 percent of the time.

• *Work to identify "bids" when your partner expresses them—both the explicit ones and the subtler ones. As often as possible, respond to your partner in a positive way when they seek your attention.*

Celebrate Good News

Psychologists define *capitalization* as celebrating someone's good news—putting an exclamation point on another's accomplishment or success. Nobody wants to feel great about some piece of news only to get a half-interested response from their partner—you want them to be more excited than you are. While it is far from surprising that people like to be celebrated, it turns out that how couples handle the *good* times may be as important as how they weather the bad ones.

In one study, seventy-nine dating couples answered questions about the strength of their relationship and taped interviews in which they discussed both positive and negative life events. Two months later, the well-being of each relationship was assessed, including whether the couple was still together. How participants responded to positive events was found to be more closely related to the strength of their relationships than discussions about negative events.

In another study, researchers found by observing newlywed couples over a two-year period that positive perceptions of capitalization were related to higher ratings of marital satisfaction for both husbands and wives.

• *Make a big deal about good news. Celebrate small daily wins in addition to major promotions or successes. If you are in a new relationship, celebrating positive events can increase intimacy and build a strong foundation for your relationship.*

Celebrate Tough Times, Too

While celebrating good news is beneficial, the way that you interpret rocky times is also key to a happy relationship. The practice of framing difficulties in one's relationship in terms of how it brought you and your partner closer together, rather than as a sign you might be incompatible, has been found to be a key predictor of relationship success. It's a concept psychologists call "glorifying the struggle" and there is evidence to back up the assertion that it works.

In one survey, 200 college students who were either in a relationship or had recently ended one answered questions about their relationship satisfaction, trajectory, and feelings of loneliness. The study found that respondents who tended to agree that marriage is difficult, but worth the effort—that is, who glorified the struggle—described higher levels of relationship satisfaction. By glorifying their struggles, the subjects were able to discuss how the couple worked together to overcome obstacles and focus on the relationship's "ability to survive."

• *Don't ignore relationship challenges. Embrace them and even elevate them as a normal, healthy part of a successful long-term relationship. Celebrate getting through a difficult patch.*

ARGUE BETTER

"Conflictual discussions are not themselves a problem, but a natural way people sometimes try to resolve problems. What matters is that people effectively calibrate their manner of speaking to one another in a manner that is appropriate for the topic and the partner. Some problems are ultimately minor in the grand scheme of things and thus there are no real benefits to behaving in oppositional ways that can be upsetting. Also, some people are more easily upset than others and thus more oppositional approaches can be riskier."

–James McNulty, professor of psychology, Florida State University

Get More Sleep

Unhappy with your relationship? Your sleep habits might be to blame. A University of Arizona study of twenty-nine heterosexual couples found that men who reported better sleep gave more positive ratings to their relationship the next day. Interestingly, women who reported negative interactions with their partners during the day reported poorer sleep that night.

EMBRACE "ACR"

"Shelly Gable, a professor at the University of California, Santa Barbara, uses the term active constructive responding, *or ACR, to describe the way to cultivate more life satisfaction–higher positive emotions and greater relationship well-being. There are four ways to respond to others' good news, and only one of these four builds stronger relationships. The other three actually break down the relationship.*

1 A passive constructive response *is brief and often distracted. It might involve a 'that's great,' but you turn your attention away from your partner; it lacks connection.*

2 A passive destructive response *ignores the event completely, hijacks the content, and turns the conversation to yourself.*

3 An active destructive response *takes the wind right out of their sails and highlights what might be wrong or worrisome about the good news.*

4 An active constructive response *(ACR) shows genuine interest by asking simple questions to help your partner savor the good news. Not only are you letting your partner experience the joy of the event, but your shared experience is a happiness multiplier."*

–Lorrie Peniston, psychotherapist

Friends' Relationships Are Important, Too

Divorce can be contagious. A team of researchers led by Rose McDermott of Brown University conducted a longitudinal study on how a person's social network can impact his or her relationship. Looking at data for thousands of people over three decades, they found that individuals were 75 percent more likely to become divorced if a friend got divorced, and 33 percent more likely to do so if a friend of a friend did. All told, the findings suggested that if a close friend or family member divorces, your chances of divorcing your partner increase by 16 percent.

· *Help your friends strengthen their own marriages. Plan couples' activities together and speak positively about friends' partners.*

Raise Your Credit Score

Financial difficulties are one of the biggest challenges a relationship can face. And as it happens, your credit score can be a pretty good predictor of your marriage's chance of survival. A study by researchers from UCLA, the Brookings Institution, and the Federal Reserve Board found that the lower a person's credit score, the more likely his or her marriage will end in divorce. They went so far as to put it in numbers: For every 105-point increase in your credit score, there is a corresponding 32 percent drop in your likelihood of divorcing. So now you have one more reason to pay off that Visa.

Create a Division of Labor

Who did the dishes last? What about the vacuuming? Chores are a complex work arrangement that if managed well can encourage cohesiveness in a household, but can create the opposite if managed poorly. In a Pew Research poll, sharing household chores was rated in the top three issues associated with a successful marriage (after faithfulness and good sex). UCLA researchers looked into exactly how these issues affected marital satisfaction. They found that on average, men spent 18 percent of their time doing housework and handled just one third of household tasks, while women took on 67 percent of household tasks while spending 22 percent of their time on housework.

It turned out there was greater conflict between couples who failed to lay out explicit terms of who was responsible for what than between those who made these distinctions clear. Ambiguity led to one person having to ask the other to pull their weight, to feelings of resentment, and to criticism of one another's performance of their tasks. The researchers concluded that the best way to avoid these conflicts is through "clear and equitable models" that reduce the need for partners to manage one another's chores. In turn, couples can "fulfill their household duties with the knowledge that the partner will not in fact overstep established boundaries."

• *Lay out clear responsibilities—you do the dishes, your spouse does the cooking, and you swap the vacuuming every other weekend.*

Rethink What You're Getting from Sex

Sex feels great—but that's not the only reason it's great. While pleasure is an important component of a healthy sex life, studies have shown that over time, a relationship succeeds when your attention is on your partner's needs and on creating intimacy between you both.

A team of researchers examining the relationship behavior of 128 couples found that men who approached sex as a means of gaining self-affirmation actually reported lower sexual satisfaction and fewer orgasms during sex. Couples who sought to increase intimacy and fulfill one another's needs expressed greater satisfaction with their sex lives.

• *Put your attention on your partner's needs, and you'll end up enjoying sex more.*

SEEK SIMILAR SPENDING HABITS

"Our work suggests tightwads would probably be better off financially and psychologically by marrying other tightwads. Spendthrifts appear to be happier, though less financially stable, when married to other spendthrifts. Pairing with your financial opposite can be fun and interesting at first, especially for tightwads, who have a hard time spending on their own. But over time, the stakes get higher—you have to jointly make decisions about things like houses, cars, and kids. There are more and more opportunities for arguments, blame, second-guessing, and regret.

"But if you're already married to your opposite, maintaining separate bank accounts might help. We're investigating this now in a field experiment with newlyweds, where we've randomly assigned them to maintain joint or separate accounts."

–Scott Rick, associate professor of marketing,
Ross School of Business, University of Michigan

Say "We"

That simple two-letter word can make a big impact on the health of your love life. A group of researchers at the University of California,

Berkeley reviewed fifteen-minute videotaped conversations between 154 married couples, and found that the use of personal pronouns such as "we," "us," and "our" were linked with positive behaviors such as affection and lower frequency of negative behaviors such as anger.

Turn On a Sappy Romance

We've all seen our share of corny romance movies, where the two beautiful people at first can't stand each other but are locked in a passionate embrace by the time the credits roll. It can all seem a bit unrealistic. But in fact, watching such elevated versions of intimate relationships can have a positive effect on your own romance.

Through an online survey, researchers asked 275 participants about their romantic expectations, beliefs, and experiences, as well as their level of commitment to their current partner. They found that the expression of romantic beliefs had a positive impact on relationship satisfaction. In other words, if we operate with a positive, even idealistic view of relationships, then we may approach our relationship in ways that strengthen the connection. And those who endorsed romantic beliefs were not found to be more likely to suffer unmet relationship expectations. The researchers suggested this might be because "romantic beliefs lead individuals to approach a relationship in a way that fosters positive outcomes." For example, if you believe your partner to be your soul mate, you're more likely to overlook a given disagreement or temporary annoyance.

· *Read a romance or watch a movie about gorgeous people falling in love. Idealizing relationships is likely to strengthen your own.*

Put On Those Rose-Colored Glasses

As we said, idealization is healthy. A longitudinal study of 200 couples recruited when they obtained marriage licenses found that those who maintain heightened views about their partners' positive qualities tended to remain happier longer.

The couples who participated in the study were surveyed twice a year for three years to assess their relationship qualities and marriage satisfaction; they were also asked questions about their own positive traits. Researchers determined who idealized their partner by comparing partner responses about themselves and each other. They found that couples in which one person indicated that their partner possessed positive, idealistic qualities and the other person did not indicate seeing those qualities within themselves—what the researchers called "illusions"—maintained higher levels of marital satisfaction longer.

· *Don't be afraid to put your partner on a pedestal and idealize the things you most admire about him or her.*

Punch Up Your "How We Met" Story

"How'd you guys meet?" might not seem like a complicated question, but it holds a great deal of insight into the strength of a couple's relationship. That was among the findings in a classic study of fifty-two couples in which each pair discussed the history of their relationship including their first impressions of one another. The researchers rated each for positive and negative elements and were able to predict—with 94 percent accuracy—whether the couple would stay together or divorce. In telling their story, the couples who were more reserved or negative were more likely to break up within three years, while the couples who were more passionate and expansive were more likely to stay together. (They were also more likely to display marital satisfaction and better problem solving.)

This extended beyond just the "how we met" story, and also covered questions such as "What types of things did you do together [when you were first dating]?" and "Tell me about your wedding." Couples with strong, positive, energizing memories of these early years are able to draw on these memories when the relationship hits a rough patch.

· Discuss early memories with your partner and the way that you met. Establish a passionate baseline for your relationship and shared story.

Maintain Friendships Outside the Marriage

Many married people describe their spouse as their best friend. That's wonderful—as long as they're not your only friend. A number of studies back up the fact that a relationship is healthier when the partners maintain friendships and hobbies outside of it. One study of 123 couples by researchers at the University of Maryland School of Social Work found that healthy couple friendships can add to a marriage in a number of ways: Couple friends increase partners' attraction to each other, give individuals the opportunity to see how other couples interact, and provide a greater understanding of men and women more broadly.

Change Up Date Night

Keeping a relationship fresh goes a long way toward keeping it happy. A researcher at the State University of New York at Stony Brook found that participating in novel activities enhanced the quality of a relationship. One experiment instructed a group of middle-aged couples to spend ninety minutes per week doing "exciting" activities—such as hiking, dancing, or attending a show—unlike what they typically did.

After ten weeks, these participants were compared to a group of couples who had been instructed to just do pleasant and familiar activities, like going to a movie or out to dinner. The "exciting" couples exhibited a much higher level of marital satisfaction.

These effects may be rooted in chemistry—specifically the release of dopamine and norepinephrine, which pop into a person's brain as they enjoy these new "self-expanding activities."

• *Try something new for date night. Create relationship missions that push you to get out of your comfort zone as a couple. Take an art class, go skydiving, or just take a road trip somewhere you've never been before.*

Keep a Journal Handy

Many people can't remember what they did last week, let alone six months ago. But researchers have found that a great sense of joy can be gained from jotting down daily activities in a journal—and from revisiting these moments at a later date. Harvard researchers found that when people recorded daily events and were asked to review them months later, they felt the experience to be both interesting and pleasurable. In one of four experiments, participants created a "time capsule," responding to nine prompts that captured recent conversations, songs they just listened to, an inside joke, or a recent photo. They predicted how curious they would be at a later date to see what they had written down; three months later they rated how surprising or meaningful they found each jotting. Participants were consistently more curious to see what they had written than they expected they would be.

In another study, participants noted their activities on Valentine's Day as well as on another, unremarkable February day, writing down how curious they would expect to feel upon rereading their account of each day. Again, they underestimated how interested they would be about reading of their mundane day. While we document birthdays, weddings, and other big events, it turns out that regular boring days are plenty exciting in hindsight, too.

· Incorporate a shared journal into your relationship, where each partner can jot down memories as they happen, to be revisited whenever you like.

Make Time for Sex

You probably aren't having enough sex. An Australian survey of more than 6,500 men and women found that 54 percent of men and 42 percent of women were unhappy with the frequency of sex in their relationship—and those who were unhappy with the frequency of sex were more likely to report lower levels of relationship satisfaction. The study's lead author, Anthony Smith, professor of public health and deputy director of the Australian Research Center in Sex, Health and Society at La Trobe University in Melbourne, told *The New York Times* that couples may need to set aside time for sex just as they do for meals, work, and other activities. As he put it, "If people value sex as an important part of their relationship, and almost everybody does, then they need to put sex higher up the priority list."

· If you aren't having sex at least a couple times a week, talk to your partner about why and maybe set a schedule of certain nights you will make time for intimacy. It may seem the opposite of sexy to plan getting it on, but if the alternative is a sexless marriage, it's worth it.

5

Happy at Home

*"Home is the place where, when you have to go there,
they have to take you in."*

**–ROBERT FROST,
"THE DEATH OF THE HIRED MAN"**

Your home is an extension of yourself. What you put in it and how others perceive it inspire as much second-guessing and anxiety as any other aspect of your personality. There's a reason those HGTV shows are so addictive. Every detail of your home not only says something about who you are, but it's something you have to live with every day—and it's likely affecting your well-being in ways you don't even realize. Neuroscientists and psychologists are increasingly finding evidence for what interior designers and architects have always known: Your environment impacts your happiness.

But figuring out the ways in which it does so, and how to create a home that maximizes your satisfaction and enjoyment, is easier said than done. Anyone who has spent a few hours at the hardware store deciding between two hundred shades of light blue paint knows that decisions about interior design can be very personal and surprisingly complicated. Should you tap into some life-changing magic by cleaning up your clutter, or will you get more joy by leaving your stuff all over the place? Is fêng shui the way? Does *hygge* hold the answers?

Here we look at some science-backed hacks to bring more joy into your home, from what you put on your walls to the shape of the walls themselves; from the texture of your living room furniture to the type of light in your bedroom.

Brighten Up

Feeling down? Turn on some lights—or at least turn them up. In three separate studies, researchers at the University of Toronto and China's Sun Yat-sen University found a correlation between people's feelings of hopelessness and their perception of room lighting. During a fourth study, participants indicated greater feelings of hopelessness when in a darker room.

Another study of 988 people from four different countries found that those living closer to the equator had more consistent psychological moods compared to those farther north, where light varied significantly throughout the year. In those more northern countries, subjects' moods were found to be at their lowest when lighting felt too dark and at their highest when respondents felt lighting was "just right"; they then declined when lighting was felt to be too bright.

If you're feeling overwhelmed with life, brighter lighting may help alleviate negative emotions, and potentially restore positive feelings.

· *Add a few more lamps around the house and increase the wattage of the bulbs in them. Use multiple sources of lighting and dimming switches for ceiling lights.*

Beware Blue Light

There's little that's as effective at boosting mood as natural light.

Studies have found that exposure to natural light throughout the day is more likely to improve your mood, help you sleep better, and better your quality of life as compared to artificial light. A key reason natural light is so healthy, particularly for your sleep, is its impact on melatonin production, which contributes to both your sense of drowsiness when it's time to sleep and how alert you are during the day. The pineal gland that produces melatonin is highly sensitive to light: It's triggered by darkness or dim light and suppressed by bright lights—including artificial "blue" light from smartphones, tablets, and energy-efficient bulbs.

And, it turns out, this blue light can trick your body into thinking that it's daytime when you should be sleeping, leading to disruptions in your sleep and causing all types of emotional and physical trouble. As a Harvard Medical School newsletter noted, "Blue wavelengths—which are beneficial during daylight hours because they boost attention, reaction times, and mood—seem to be the most disruptive at night." And with smartphones and tablets everywhere, including the bedroom, we are more exposed than ever to these blue wavelengths.

· *Keep mobile devices out of the bedroom, especially at night. Use a dim red bulb—which is least likely to depress melatonin production—for your reading light.*

Create a Fake Sun

In the morning, it's a different story. If your home, or just your bedroom, doesn't get a lot of natural light, you'll be happy to hear that even just simulating the sun can benefit your well-being. A team of Swiss researchers tested a group of people over a forty-eight-hour period using three different light conditions: a blue monochromatic LED, a dawn-simulating light, and a dim light. The researchers measured subjects' mood and well-being—including melatonin and cortisol levels—every two hours. They found that the light simulating the dawn had a positive effect on cognition, mood, and well-being far more than the other lights.

• *Your body is surprisingly gullible. If your bedroom doesn't get much natural light, pick up a dawn-simulating lamp to fake yourself into thinking the sun is shining in.*

BRING IN THE SUNLIGHT

"Our research looked at office employees and how much natural light they had. We found that those who had natural light throughout the day slept forty-six minutes per night more on average than those who did not. And there was another puzzling finding: they tended to spend more time outside in their free time than those without natural light. I don't know exactly how to explain that, but it may be that those who had natural light felt more energetic and were keen to do more activities at the end of the day."

–Mohamed Boubekri, professor, Illinois School of Architecture,
University of Illinois at Urbana-Champaign

Place Your Desk Sideways to the Window

But to get the most out of the natural light coming through your window, don't face it head-on. A study looking at the impact of sunlight on a person's emotional state found that the amount of sunlight penetrating a room had a significant impact on subjects' feelings of relaxation—when they were sitting sideways to the window. The level of relaxation decreased when the person was facing directly toward the window or had their back to it.

Be Messy—in Creative Places

We've all heard the stories of how creative types embrace their messy side, but researchers have also found empirical evidence that messiness can help you think more imaginatively. A trio of experiments dove into this topic, comparing how participants performed when asked to complete a creative task in a cluttered room versus an organized room.

In the first, participants were randomly assigned to either a messy room (with paper and books strewn about) or an orderly room (with all those papers and books carefully stacked and organized) and asked to complete a puzzle. In the second experiment, participants were asked to complete the Remote Associates Test (RAT), designed to identify creative ability, in similar conditions. Finally, a different set of participants was asked to complete a drawing of their choosing in either a messy room, a cleared room, or an orderly room; the drawings were then scored for creativity by a panel of judges. The results were consistent across the all three experiments: Those in the messy room completed the puzzle fastest, scored highest on the creativity test, and earned the best marks from the drawing-judging panel.

· In areas where you get creative—your home office, workshop, or (for you kinky types) bedroom—let things get messy. But remember that a little clutter goes a long way: The researchers warn that excessive messiness can cause sensory overload and mental shutdown.

But Skip the Abstract Art

Beauty is in the eye of the beholder, especially when it comes to the sort of art you put on your walls. If you're finding yourself feeling a bit stressed at home, you might want to rethink how you're decorating your walls. Architecture professor Roger Ulrich, who studied how hospital design affects patient well-being, found that art on the walls generally elicits positive feelings and keeps patients' attention— even distracting them from discomfort or worries. But not all art proved healthy: While patients found landscapes and nature scenes pleasing, in interviews patients reported feeling disturbed by abstract art.

Ulrich dug into this trend further, and found that seven paintings had actually been targets of physical attacks over the previous seven years, with five of those having been attacked more than once. All seven were works of abstract art, and all were eventually removed.

* *If you're finding yourself feeling stressed or itching to attack your wall, change the artwork on it.*

Warm Up Your Walls

Add some excitement to your life by changing up your home's paint colors. While there have been numerous studies on the relationship between color and mood, a big area to consider is whether the color is warm (such as red or orange), cool (blue or violet), or achromatic (neutral grays, black, or white).

To figure out how people respond to these different color temperatures, researchers developed two "virtual living rooms" and varied the placement of the window, furniture, and shelving units in them. Participants were shown three pictures of each room, each with a different type of coloring (warm, cool, or achromatic).

Warm colors were consistently rated as more stimulating and exciting; cool colors were considered more spacious, restful, calm, and peaceful, while achromatic colors had the lowest positive ratings.

• *Boost the "excitement" of rooms like kitchens and home gyms, where you'll want to have high energy, with warm colors. Go with cooler options for places where a more calming feeling would work best, such as a bedroom or study. Skip the achromatic colors altogether.*

Raise the Roof

If you're working on a project that requires creativity, seek out a space in your home where the ceiling is at its highest—or maybe just go outside. A pair of marketing professors conducted a trio of experiments looking at individuals' responses to rooms that were identical except for ceiling height. They found that higher ceilings induced a greater sense of freedom in individuals—not to mention sharper memory.

Love Those Curves

Does your home or office put you on edge? It might be that it has too many sharp edges. People find curved surfaces more pleasing than sharp ones: When presented with 140 grayscale images of various items (such as watches and cooling fans), participants expressed a preference for those with curved edges. This tendency was also true for meaningless patterns drawn with either sharp lines or curved lines. So if you're picking out a desk or dresser, look for one with rounded edges. Extra bonus: Curved edges hurt a lot less when you bump into them.

Place a Notepad and Trash Can Near the Mirror

Sounds like a weird tip, but hear me out. Researchers have found that by giving thoughts a physical form, as through writing, people are able to throw their thoughts away, literally.

In the study, participants were randomly assigned to write either positive thoughts or negative thoughts about their bodies. They were then randomly asked to either throw the written thoughts into a wastebasket, or check their writing for any grammatical errors. Afterward, they completed a questionnaire to determine their attitude toward their bodies. The thoughts—whether positive or negative—that had been "thrown away" were found to have had less of an impact.

So throwing them out is an effective way to get rid of negative thoughts, but a similar logic works for internalizing positive thoughts. During a second experiment by the same researchers, participants were told to pull out the page on which they'd written thoughts about their body image, fold it, and put it in their pockets, while members of a control group were told to just fold down the corners of the paper so it could be identified later if needed. All were then asked to fill out a questionnaire about health and diet. Participants who had kept their thoughts safe responded more positively or more negatively (depending on the type of thought written down) than the control group.

• *Having a bad hair day? Worried that top makes you look fat? Cut down on these negative thoughts by placing a notebook and trash can in front of your mirror, so you can "throw away" negative thoughts about yourself in the moment—or choose to keep the positive thoughts in your pocket.*

If You Build It . . .

You get more joy from the things in your home that you make yourself. That was the finding of a group of researchers from Harvard, Duke, and Tulane Universities, who found that when a group of subjects exerted effort to produce three different products (IKEA storage boxes, origami, and Lego models), it increased the value that they placed on those objects.

The researchers found that this tendency to place value on items that took effort to assemble held true not just for individuals who considered themselves do-it-yourselfers. Participants who hardly considered themselves handy also placed greater value on what they'd made. There was also a tendency to overvalue the items that participants had built themselves—placing *more* importance on the built items than on those made by experts or machines.

· *Instead of just buying a piece of furniture, try to build it yourself (even if IKEA does most of the work for you). Add a few self-made items around your house, whether by putting knickknacks on shelves or hanging art you've made on the wall.*

Get Some Flowers

Flowers can do amazing things for your well-being. In one study conducted by researchers from Rutgers and La Salle Universities, three experiments were used to explore the relationship between flowers and mood. During one of the experiments, participants received a delivery of either flowers or another "gift" (fruit basket or candles) to their homes. Experimenters measured the initial response of the participant (specifically their smile) and conducted interviews later on.

All of the participants who received flowers smiled upon the delivery. Furthermore, researchers found during the follow-up interviews that participants who had received the flowers tended to put them in areas where they could be enjoyed by others, and reported more positive social interactions throughout the day in comparison to the groups who had received a different gift. So get to a florist already!

GET A PET

"Pet owners tend to have greater self-esteem, tend to be in better physical shape, and tend to be less lonely than non-pet owners. When people have recently experienced a social rejection, thinking about their pet improves their well-being to the same extent that thinking about their best friend does.

"Obviously, the social support you get from your pet is perceived–your dog or cat isn't interested in having a conversation with you–but when you feel like it cares about you and is attentive to you, you get a lot of the same benefits that you would from having a conversation or a social interaction.

"We've never found differences [in emotional benefits] between dogs and cats. The primary difference is the extent to which you anthropomorphize the pet: If you view your iguana as having human-like compassion and qualities, it's as good as a golden retriever. It's all in the mind of the owner."

–Allen McConnell

Enjoy the View

Numerous studies have found evidence of the happiness-boosting benefits of spending time outdoors and looking at natural surroundings. But if you don't have time for a hike, simply looking at trees can help reduce stress. A study of prisoners found that those who had views from their cells of the surrounding landscape suffered stress-related illnesses less frequently than prisoners who did not have these views. Another study of patients recovering from gall bladder surgery showed that those who could view trees from their beds improved more rapidly than those who could not.

In addition to helping overcome stress, viewing trees helps to sharpen people's attention. In a comparison of college students, those who had views of nature from their dorms felt less mental fatigue than those who only saw parking lots and sidewalks.

· *Try to find a place with a view of trees and nature. Take a minute or two each day to appreciate the view.*

When You Feel Bad, Reach Out and Touch Something

You're more sensitive to touch when in a bad mood. Through a series of five separate experiments, a pair of marketing researchers demonstrated that those in "negative affective states" (bad moods) were especially sensitive to the feel of a product (skin lotion, in the case of the experiment), describing it in tactile terms, rather than the visual terms they used to describe it when in a positive mood.

The heightened sensitivity led participants to feel "a more positive hedonic response from the enhanced tactile stimulation," as the researchers put it. In other words, the worse you feel, the more sensitive your touch. The researchers suggested that this grows out of our evolutionary biological functioning: When we are injured, hurt, or vulnerable, there is a biological need to find protection, warmth, and security.

• Keep soft objects on hand and create tactile comfort. After a hard day, you will be extra sensitive to them and they may even turn your bad mood around.

Create a "Relaxation Room"

When feeling stressed or anxious, turning on calming music can be as relaxing as a massage. Researchers studied a group of sixty-eight participants who suffered from feelings of anxiety. They randomly assigned them to three treatment conditions: therapeutic massage, thermotherapy control group (in which warm heating pads and towels were placed on various parts of the body), and relaxing room control group (where they listened to relaxing music through a CD player). Participants attended weekly one-hour sessions a total of ten times within twelve weeks.

All three groups showed significant improvements on anxiety tests following treatments, but researchers did not find that massage or thermotherapy was more effective than simply relaxing and enjoying music. They hypothesized that the common elements to the three groups—a safe environment, the opportunity to take time out from life, and encouragement to practice deep breathing—may have been responsible for the improvements.

• Skip the $200 massage and just download an album of relaxing music. Create a relaxation room in your home that can serve as a refuge from the rest of your busy life and household—even if it's just for half an hour.

Turn Off the TV

The warm glow of the television might actually be bumming you out. A pair of researchers looking at what happy people do differently from unhappy people reviewed data from the General Social Survey (GSS), which tracks changing social characteristics and attitudes through personal interviews over a span of thirty-five years. These researchers looked at information from more than 45,000 people on what they did in their free time. Happiness was rated based on respondents' self-reports.

They found that happy people reported being more engaged in social activities, religion, and newspaper reading (okay, so the research is a few years old). The only activity that correlated negatively with happiness was television viewing—meaning that people who watched more hours of television in an average sitting were more likely to report that they were unhappy. While this research does not prove that television viewing causes unhappiness (unhappy people may use television to escape from reality), it does show a correlation between the two.

· *Get away from your TV and call some friends. Review your viewing habits, and cut back on the hours spent streaming.*

Get a Savings Jar

In Chapter 3, we discussed how spending money on life experiences, rather than on material objects, leads to greater levels of happiness. But whether buying things or experiences, making a purchase has been found to generate three distinct types of happiness: anticipatory happiness, momentary happiness, and afterglow happiness.

You can increase anticipatory happiness in your home by using a visual tool—a savings jar—to remind yourself of the purchase goal you are working toward, whether it's to buy a new pair of shoes or book a vacation. The jar does not need to be large—this study looked at purchases of around twenty dollars—but it should note what the money will be going toward, to maximize your anticipatory happiness as well as to help you focus on your goal.

· *Maximize the joy you get from making a purchase by putting a savings jar in your house and note what the money will be going toward.*

Reconsider That Open-Concept Kitchen

Open-concept kitchens are all the rage, but if you're trying to cut back on how much you're eating in order to enhance your overall wellness and health, you might want to add back a few of those walls. Research has found that dining areas' floor plans have an impact on the amount of food we consume. In a comparison study of open and closed floor plans, an architecture researcher and a design researcher found that closed areas resulted in fewer servings being consumed, presumably because diners could not see the extra food that was available.

· *Add a divider screen, if not a wall, between your kitchen and dining areas.*

Move Closer to Work

A long commute can take a serious toll on your level of happiness. Research in Sweden found that happiness ratings decreased the longer the commute. It was also found that commuting by walking or biking was correlated to higher happiness ratings than having to rely on public transit or a car.

· *When choosing where to purchase or rent your home, give extra weight to the length of the commute.*

Rent Instead of Buy

The question "Should I rent or should I buy?" has tormented people for decades, with no easy answer. Considerations ranging from personal budget to family size to location shape how one comes to a decision. But for those looking to enhance their level of happiness, the answer seems pretty clear: Stick with a rental. The *Telegraph* conducted a survey of 5,800 United Kingdom citizens to investigate whether people were happier renting or owning their homes. The survey questions focused on how financial circumstances contributed to happiness and stress levels, and the results showed that those who rented a detached home were the least stressed.

Even though the survey found that people who rent their homes tended to spend a greater portion of their finances on housing, the survey results also showed that homeowners were just as likely to list money as their biggest concern. The survey also found that people renting a room or a detached house were more likely than those who owned their homes to believe they had a good work-life balance. Not only that, renters reported enjoying relaxing at home more than homeowners, who tended to put traveling as one of their primary keys to happiness.

· Consider simplifying your life and reducing stress by just renting your place.

Reduce, Reuse, and Smile

Going green is not just good for the planet—it has also been found to put those who do it into a better mood. The Happiness Research Institute of the Danish Ministry of the Environment found a link between behaviors that benefit the environment and individual happiness. Those who instituted household practices such as using recycling bins, composting, or installing water-saving faucets or energy-saving appliances reported an uptick in their level of happiness. Data on fourteen European countries showed that people who recycle are happier on average than those who do not (by about 0.2 on a three-point scale). One report found that living more sustainably—for example, riding a bike to work instead of driving a car, or waiting to start a load of laundry until the machine is full—promotes a more fulfilling and happier life. A study of residents of fourteen Chinese cities showed that those who work to reduce waste and save energy score higher on life satisfaction than those who are mildly engaged or unengaged in sustainable behaviors.

The researchers suggest that this occurs because of evolutionary factors: We experience feelings of pleasure whenever we engage in activities that increase the likelihood of species survival. These behaviors can also lead to greater feelings of personal accomplishment and feeling more connected to our communities as a whole. Or maybe we're just glad not to have so much junk around the house.

· *Pick up a recycling bin, start composting, or do something else to help out Mother Nature.*

6

HƏPPY iN FRiENDShiP

"The ornament of a house is the friends who frequent it."

–RALPH WALDO EMERSON

Your friends are the people you call to waste an afternoon, catch a movie, or grab a few too many drinks on a random weeknight. They are also the ones who see you at your extremes, among the first people you tell about a big accomplishment or who help you deal with frustration or loss. When you decide to try something risky—a major career move, a new dance move—your social network is the safety net that catches you if things go sideways (though they also have permission to tease you when they do). It's no wonder these people have such an impact on your emotional well-being. Researchers have found that having a happy friend can boost your own probability of happiness by 15.3 percent, and by even more if they live near you. Studies indicate that those with good friends are resilient to negative events and even live longer. Your group of friends—its size, its makeup, and how you interact with one another—shapes your happiness in ways large and small.

So what are the secrets to creating a happy social circle and infusing your friendships with fun? This chapter suggests some answers, drawing on what researchers have learned about developing emotional intelligence, making new friends, and cultivating lasting, happy friendships.

150 Is the Magic Number

The greatest number of meaningful relationships a person can maintain is about 150. That number was famously set by British anthropologist Robin Dunbar (and the number of meaningful friends we can have has duly been named "Dunbar's number"). He came to this while studying how primates groom one another, extending to humans the hypothesis that the average size of a species' brain reflects the average size and complexity of the social group it lives within.

For humans, Dunbar's math indicated that we could have between 100 and 200 people—so 150, on average—in our social group. This is the number of casual friends you can expect to retain before you start forgetting names or from where you know someone.

The number 150 is not just a matter of speculation. Dunbar and his colleagues found evidence of it far and wide. In most armies, even ancient ones, company sizes have ranged between 130 and 150 people. Communities such as the Amish, Mennonites, and Hutterites generally number about 150 and split once they exceed that amount. In one experiment, the average number of Christmas cards a UK household sent out reached a total of about 150 people per person sending them. Even as social media has seen the number of "connections" grow into the thousands (more on that in Chapter 8), the number of substantive friendships we can handle remains surprisingly consistent.

Layer Up

This magic number can also be separated into distinct layers or concentric circles, which Dunbar calls "circles of acquaintanceship." This roughly breaks down to a small circle closest to the center that represents our approximately five closest friends, followed by the next group of fifteen, followed by a fifty-person layer representing individuals we see most often in person or at parties. The 150 layer is good friends and family, many of whom may be geographically distant, then a 500-person layer of acquaintances, and finally a 1,500-person layer that Dunbar characterizes as the typical size of the tribe.

· *Review your five-, fifteen-, and fifty-person circles: Who are your closest friends? Who should be moved into an inner circle?*

A FACEBOOK CONNECTION IS NOT A FRIEND

"Young people using Facebook and spending their time online are very much connected, but they experience more and more loneliness. In a way, they don't understand the importance of real friendship, of intimacy. When you are all the time promoting yourself and trying to get the world excited about how happy you are or how well you're doing and don't differentiate between different types of friends, you don't get intimacy—real friendship demands being yourself, not selling your happiness and selling what you want to be. They can be connected in the morning and all day long, but they don't get the benefits of real friendship. This feeling that you don't need to invest the time anymore, that you could have a friend just like that, it's an illusion that we're efficient."

–Yair Amichai-Hamburger, director of the Research Center for Internet Psychology, Sammy Ofer School of Communications at the Interdisciplinary Center in Israel, and author of *Internet Psychology: The Basics*

Seek Out Happy Friends—and Acquaintances

Like a common cold, yawning, and much else, happiness is contagious. Surrounding yourself with happy people has been found to help boost your own level of subjective well-being. But beyond that, the people your friends spend time with also can impact your own happiness. Researchers from Harvard and the University of California, San Diego came to this finding through the surveys of the 4,739 respondents to the famed Framingham Heart Study. In addition to details about their personal habits and cardiovascular health, the residents of Framingham, Massachusetts, who filled out the questionnaire offered answers about their happiness and social contacts over a period of decades. Cross-referencing these responses, the researchers found that the people who reported being happy formed "clusters," with those reporting the highest levels of happiness located at the center of those clusters.

They crunched the numbers to come up with specific probabilities of happiness with which each level of connection is associated. Specifically, your likelihood of happiness rises:

- 15.3 percent if a family member or close friend is happy
- 9.8 percent if friends of your family members or friends are happy
- 5.6 percent if friends of those friends of your family members or friends are happy

· *Add more happy people to your social circles. Even having happy people in your life tangentially boosts the likelihood that you will find happiness.*

Get Closer

When it comes to boosting your happiness by surrounding yourself with happy people, proximity counts. The same research drawing on the Framingham Heart Study found that living within a mile of a friend who has become happier increases the probability that you will be happy by 25 percent. A next-door neighbor who goes from unhappy to happy can increase your happiness by 34 percent.

Smell a Happy Person

This may be part of the reason proximity enhances happiness. Our sweat sends all kinds of signals, from fear to sexual arousal, that another person can sense. And it turns out positive emotions like happiness can also be conveyed through scents—and boost the emotions of those near enough to pick up on them.

Psychology researchers from Utrecht University in the Netherlands tested this theory by getting twelve male participants to sit in a warm, dark room. There, they watched videos meant to inspire different emotional responses (the catchy "Bear Necessities" song from Disney's *The Jungle Book*, boring weather reports, or frightening scenes from the film *The Shining*), sweating into sterile pads for each. Thirty-six women then sniffed each type of sweat (okay, this got pretty gross), and assessed the "pleasantness and intensity" of the sweat. Though neither the researchers nor the subjects knew which sweat was which, the subjects who sniffed the "happy sweat" exhibited more cheerful expressions and a more positive mood than those taking in the other types of sweat, when controlled for other variables.

According to the researchers, this indicates "behavior synchronization" between the sweater and the smeller. Of course, going around and smelling happy people might not be the most efficient way to boost your mood, but as researcher Gün Semin put it, "This suggests that somebody who is happy will infuse others in their vicinity with happiness. In a way, happiness sweat is somewhat like smiling—it is infectious."

• *Surround yourself with upbeat people, and their presence is likely to trigger a sense of happiness in you.*

Spend More Time Together

Familiarity breeds friendship. Experiments by a team of researchers put two strangers together, encouraging them to interact for varying amounts of time. The more two people interacted with each other, the more attracted they were to one another. According to the psychologists conducting the research, three processes contributed to the dynamic: a sense of responsiveness in the other person, greater comfort and satisfaction during the interaction, and a perception of knowing the other person.

• *Showing up is 80 percent (or thereabouts) of friendship. If you want to build a friendship, make the effort to spend more time with prospective friends.*

Get Personal

In as short a time as 45 minutes, you can build a strong bond with a complete stranger. That was among the findings of research published in *Personality and Social Psychology Bulletin*, in which a group of psychology students were paired off. Researchers tasked some of the pairs to follow a series of prompts that led them to reveal personal, even intimate details about themselves, while the others just kept to light small talk. At the end, those who got more personal expressed feeling a significantly deeper connection with their partner—in approximately 30 percent of respondents, the connection was viewed as closer than their most intimate relationships. After the experiment, more than half of those in the "self-disclosure" group stayed in touch while more than one third met up and did something together.

• *Next time you are having drinks or coffee with a friend, talk about your feelings, rather than thoughts or opinions. Lasting friendships grow from getting personal.*

CULTIVATE ENGAGED CONVERSATIONS

"Active listening is an actual process that generates greater satisfaction in friendships, working relationships, family relationships, and intimate partner relationships because the outcome of active listening offers maximum support to the speaker. When individuals feel supported (especially when the friendship is forming), the rate of self-disclosure is higher. Self-disclosure, or the knowledge that you would share with new people, yields better, more immediate bonds, an outcome of which is greater satisfaction in the relationship."

–Elizabeth M. Minei, assistant professor of communications,
Baruch College, City University of New York

Less Can Be More . . .

More is not always merrier. A large group of friends says plenty about your likability, but not much about whether you're likely to be happy. Researchers have found that the quality of friendships has been most often associated with one's overall happiness, when controlled for one's personality. So as the researchers put it, even if you are someone predisposed to being happy, investing in quality friendships "still add[s] something extra to our lives and has the potential to increase one's happiness."

• *Focus on a handful of close friendships first, before trying to appeal to a large number of acquaintances.*

. . . But Acquaintances Are Key

While quality friendships are the most important for one's happiness, studies have also found that the people we just kind of know—what scientists call "weak ties"—can play an important role in boosting our happiness. One study examined the relationships between students in a classroom and concluded that those who had more daily interactions with other classmates who weren't their close friends were happier and had a greater feeling of belonging than those with a limited social circle.

The researchers suggest that we "chat with the coffee barista, work colleague, yoga classmate, and [fellow] dog owner—these interactions may contribute meaningfully to our happiness, above and beyond the contribution of interactions with our close friends and family." Additionally, while long-lasting friendships aren't always the same as high-quality friendships, researchers have found that friends you know for a long time, even if only casually, make a valuable contribution to your happiness.

Beyond that, weak ties may be good for your creativity. According to Jill Perry-Smith at Emory University's Goizueta Business School, while strong social ties have a neutral effect, weak ties bolster one's individual creativity. It is not entirely clear why this happens, but according to Perry-Smith, empirical evidence suggests that weak ties facilitate "the generation of alternatives and encourage autonomous thinking."

· *Diversify your "friend portfolio" with acquaintances, making sure "weak ties" are part of your life.*

Give . . .

Few things boost your happiness as reliably as giving. Adults with a wide range of backgrounds, cultures, and demographics report experiencing elevated levels of happiness when donating to charity or spending money on others rather than themselves. Anthropologists

TURN A WORKPLACE ACQUAINTANCE INTO A GREAT FRIEND

While it used to be the case that employers expected workers to keep their personal lives at home, it turns out that having a good friend at work can hugely benefit your productivity. Research shows that those who have good friends at the office are much more engaged and effective at their jobs. This is largely because the stakes are much higher: Letting down a boss is one thing, but disappointing a good friend is much tougher.

To get more out of work and build stronger friendships, there are three steps a workplace friendship goes through, according to Washington State University researchers Patricia Sias and Daniel Cahill. Examining nineteen close workplace friendships, they identified three phases of moving from acquaintance to almost-best friend:

❶ Acquaintance to friend, as nonworkplace topics are discussed with more frequency

❷ Friend to close friend, as they connect more closely over problems in work or life

❸ Close friend to almost-best friend, as time passes and life events strengthen the bond

The strongest fuel for creating a connection between workmates? Commiserating over work or personal problems. That vulnerability and openness is the foundation on which deep friendships are built.

· Identify a problem you and a colleague can work together to solve, or at least can commiserate over. Nothing jumpstarts a workplace friendship faster.

and evolutionary psychologists theorize that the rewarding feelings one gets from helping others have developed in order to help create prosocial and cooperative behavior among humans living and functioning together.

But it's not just adults who have been found to benefit from selfless behavior. While we think of kids as self-centered, a study of toddlers before the age of two found that they exhibited happiness when giving rather than receiving. In the experiment, each toddler received either Goldfish crackers or Teddy Grahams, and were encouraged to either enjoy them or give them to a puppet that they were told "liked treats." The treats given to the puppet were dropped into a bowl and the puppet "ate" them, making satisfied "yum" noises. The kids exhibited greater happiness when giving the treats to the puppets than when enjoying them for themselves.

· *Give a few Teddy Grahams to any treat-loving puppets you may know—and give a friend a gift or join them in a volunteer activity to get that endorphin rush of doing a good deed.*

. . . Experiences . . .

Just as experiences beat out objects when it comes to shopping for yourself, if you're looking to strengthen your friendship with a gift, go with something the friend can *do*, rather than *have*. In a study of fifty-nine pairs of friends, one person was assigned the task of purchasing a $15 gift for a buddy—either a tangible item or an experiential gift. Recipients rated the strength of their relationship with the friend before receiving the gift, then a few days after, then a week later. The experiential gifts had a stronger impact than the material gifts on the perceived strength of the friendship. Interestingly, perceived thoughtfulness and liking of the gift did not statistically impact the results; the important thing was that it was something the friends could actually experience.

. . . But Don't Be Too Generous

But while giving can boost your well-being and strengthen a friendship, being overly generous can actually damage social connections, with research showing that people-pleasers can be a serious turnoff. Researchers from Washington State University and the Desert Research Institute in Las Vegas asked subjects to play a game in which they could both contribute to and withdraw from individual or group rewards, along with a team of four other members (who were in fact computer simulations). After several transactions, the subjects could indicate how much they wanted each member to remain in the group. As might be expected, those "team members" who took more than their share from the rewards while contributing little received lower scores than those who made moderate contributions and withdrawals.

But at the same time, those who did the opposite—contributing much while taking little—were *also* selected for dismissal from the team. Through additional experiments and follow-up questions, the researchers determined that while it would seem foolish to reject someone who was willing to contribute more than their fair share, such cost-benefit analysis was tempered by "an equally strong, perhaps stronger, desire for equality of participation." The researchers suggest the reasons for this may be the competitiveness an unselfish person inspires (with others feeling obliged to give more in order to keep up) or resentment that the generous person is breaking social norms.

• *Strike a balance in your generosity. If you've bought your friend a birthday gift for three years running and they've never given you one, maybe look for another avenue for your benevolence.*

Climb the "Local Ladder"

The amount of money in your bank account and the nice things you have don't affect your level of subjective well-being as much as what your friends *think* of your bank account and nice things. Researchers have found that your life satisfaction and levels of positive or negative emotions are affected significantly by the admiration and respect you receive from your social group—the people you see face to face.

In a series of studies (including one comparing members of student groups such as sororities and ROTC organizations, and one that looked at a national sample of college kids), researchers consistently found that "sociometric status" beat out socioeconomic status as a predictor of subjective well-being. When someone rose in status among their peers, they felt happier—far more than when their income simply rose. The researchers dubbed this "the local-ladder effect."

BE PRESENT

"Being fully present in your relationships with others is key to the success of those relationships. If you're running through your mental to-do list while you're playing with your kids or 'listening' to your spouse, then you aren't really fostering the relationship."

–Holly Schiffrin, professor of psychology, University of Mary Washington (Fredericksburg, VA); coauthor of *Balancing the Big Stuff: Finding Happiness in Work, Family, and Life*

Complain with Purpose

Happy people have a specific way of complaining. Researchers looking into how happy people tend to complain surveyed 410 college

FOLLOW THE FIVE STEPS OF EMOTIONAL INTELLIGENCE

You are no doubt familiar with the concept of emotional intelligence–a person's ability to deal with their own emotions and respond to the emotions of others. It's sometimes discussed as an instinct we have intuitively. But psychologist Daniel Goleman has developed a mixed model of five competencies of emotional intelligence, which research indicates we can develop in ourselves.

❶ **Self-awareness:** Understanding your own emotions and what sets you off (by keeping a journal to track your emotions and responses throughout the day)

❷ **Self-management:** The ability to respond to these emotions and avoid overreaction or outbursts, keeping your feelings from creating trouble in your life and relationships (by breathing deeply and counting to ten when feeling stressed or angry)

❸ **Empathy:** Understanding and responding to the emotions of others (by shifting your focus to the interests and emotional needs of others)

❹ **Social/relationship skills:** The application of empathy into active behavior, forging connections with others and being persuasive when necessary (by encouraging others to talk about themselves)

❺ **Motivation:** The ability to push yourself to reach your goals (by proactively starting on a project)

Determine on which of the five steps of emotional intelligence you need the most work, and follow the accompanying tip suggested above.

students about their pet peeves with current or former relationship partners. The study found that those who complain in a more "deliberate" way—that is, with a purpose toward helping fix the thing that is causing irritation—tend to be happier. The researchers attributed this to the old buzz word, "mindfulness," suggesting that "perhaps people who are more mindful modulate the type of complaints they offer, preferring to engage in instrumental types of complaints over expressive complaints."

· *When you're about to complain, stop for at least a moment and consider how you would prefer things to be and how they could be improved, rather than simply voicing the complaint.*

Sample a Complaint Sandwich

Complaining can chip away at our level of happiness. One study found that frequent complainers suffer worse moods and experience them for longer than those who abstain from complaining. Telling someone about a personal slight or a product with which we are disappointed rarely provides the response we seek—often because we are just venting to friends or loved ones rather than going to the source of our aggravation. But science says it does not have to be this way. According to psychotherapist Guy Winch, who wrote a book about the subject, complaining with an eye toward solving problems and creating change can make venting both more satisfying and more effective.

This is best done using what Winch calls a "complaint sandwich." This begins with the "ear opener," an opening line aimed at easing the person you are speaking to into your complaint, to keep from putting them on the defensive ("Thanks for taking my call so quickly ..."). Next is the complaint (" ... but it looks like I've been overcharged on my phone bill this month"), followed by the "digestive" (a positive statement similar to the ear opener—"I'm always so happy with your service,

I hope this will be simple enough to fix"). Follow this process, and not only will the person to whom you are complaining be more likely to respond, you'll feel better in the process.

EMBARRASSMENT CAN BE GOOD

"Teasing promotes positive relationships when it is done in the spirit of play. It helps people make light of conflicts and engage in the realm of humor and lightheartedness. Embarrassment triggers prosocial tendencies in others–liking, forgiveness, trust, affection."

–Dacher Keltner, professor of psychology and codirector of the Greater Good Science Center, University of California, Berkeley

Apologize Effectively

Just as there is an effective way to complain, there is also an effective way to apologize. Not all apologies work equally well. To discern what makes the difference, a series of studies isolated three components of an apology—expressing empathy, acknowledging that social norms have been violated, and offering compensation—and examined how each component impacts the effect of the apology with the recipient.

It turned out that the apology's effectiveness was shaped by the recipient's "self-view." That is, those who tracked how much each person brought to their relationships (e.g., a coworker or boss) tended to be most impacted by offers of compensation. Those who viewed relationships as part of a larger community (such as a teammate) cared more about the recognition of how social norms were violated. The takeaway is that the most effective way to handle an apology is to be sure each apology component is included, while putting a greater focus on the one likely to matter most to that specific relationship.

For example, when apologizing to a romantic partner, empathy would be better emphasized ("I understand you're disappointed in my mistake"). For friendships, it might make more sense to focus on wider social norms.

• *When apologizing, include each essential component, but be sure to vary the balance depending on the particular relationship.*

Make Friends Feel Competent

Researchers at Northern Arizona University looked at the effect of different "friendship experiences" on the happiness of 4,382 college students to discern what kind of friendship was most likely to boost happiness. Through online surveys, the subjects were asked to assess the quality of their connection to a best friend in three areas: capitalization (whether their best friend is a good personal cheerleader); perceived mattering (whether they are important to their best friend); and satisfaction of psychological needs (whether they feel connected to their best friend, as well as feeling competent and able to be themselves around their friend). These were then analyzed in light of subjects' respective, self-reported happiness levels.

The researchers found that "needs satisfaction is the most important relationship experience" of the three when it comes to predicting a person's happiness. Drilling down deeper, they found that the most likely predictor of happiness of the three psychological needs is having a best friend who satisfies your psychological need to feel competent.

• *Seek out friends who make you feel capable and competent, and provide the same to your friends.*

FOLLOW THE RULES OF FRIENDSHIP

What makes a strong friendship? The answer would seem to vary from person to person, but back in 1984, researchers Michael Argyle and Monika Henderson pinned down some specific answers when conducting an international study on friendships that attempted to determine which rules are important for sustaining close social ties. Surveying subjects in Britain, Italy, Hong Kong, and Japan, the examiners proposed forty-three "friendship rules" to the participants, who were to answer how important each rule was to them in relation to friendship. They followed this up with studies that found differences in rule keeping between active friendships and those that had ended or lapsed, as well as with a study aimed at determining the role that the breaking of particular rules played in the dissolution of friendships. These findings pointed to six rules that made the biggest impact in the strength and continuity of friendships:

❶ Sharing news of success with the other

❷ Showing emotional support

❸ Volunteering to help in time of need

❹ Striving to make the other happy while together in company

❺ Trusting and having confidence in the other

❻ Standing up for the other in their absence

Make these rules a priority in your friendships and find ways to follow them more closely.

Don't Let a New Job Kill Old Friendships

While a new job introduces you to a new social circle, it has been found to hurt existing friendships. A longitudinal study looked at how transitioning into a job impacts individuals' social networks at three time periods, asking seventy-seven university students who were about to enter the workforce to write down up to fifty members of their social circles, detailing their interactions with each. They did the same about a year later, then another year after that.

The researchers, Donna L. Sollie and Judith L. Fischer, concluded that there is "a partial withdrawal from friends and an increase in kin contact" among those who start a new job. As subjects developed further in their careers, the number of friends in their social networks decreased, as did the amount of time they spent with those friends. At each stage the researchers examined, the friend groups included more than one-third friends who were new to the network. The researchers summarized, "being further along in one's career is likely to result in a somewhat smaller network." At the same time, the study found that respondents expressed greater commitment to remaining in their friendships as they moved further along in their careers (something that was not seen in relation to family members).

· *When starting a new job, block out time to spend with your friends, or prepare to lose some of them.*

Watch Those Drinks

While it's hardly a surprise that we drink more when out with friends, it turns out that the more friends, the more we drink. A study in Switzerland found that the number of friends present at the table has been associated with the amount one drinks. The study showed that the higher the number of friends present, the higher the number of drinks consumed per person per hour. Interestingly enough, while men generally drink more—and faster—than women, this difference becomes even greater when friends are involved.

7

Happy iN Health

"Be not sick too late, nor well too soon."

–BENJAMIN FRANKLIN

Anyone who has experienced a mildly euphoric feeling after working out for the first time in a while can appreciate the connection between physical and mental health. The two are intertwined, and often the simplest solution to a bad mood is to get up and move around. Exercise and eating the right foods don't just help you live longer and healthier; they improve your emotional state and can impact your long-term life satisfaction.

Your emotional health affects your physical health, as well. Happy people have been found to have lower heart rates (about six beats per minute slower) and stronger immune systems, and live an average of ten years longer than unhappy people, various studies have found. A rush of positive emotion has been found to reduce headaches and chest pain. And if nothing else, a hearty laugh is a simple way to burn a few calories.

This chapter outlines the scientific reasons behind these findings, with tips for how you can get both happier and healthier.

Ten Minutes Is Enough

Plenty of studies have demonstrated the connections between exercise and improved mood, reduced stress, and a greater sense of well-being. But a group of researchers sought to answer the specific question, "How much exercise is enough to feel better?" with participants taking a mood inventory before and after a quiet resting trial, then spending ten, twenty, or thirty minutes on a bicycle. Feelings of confusion, fatigue, and negative mood improved after just ten minutes of exercise. After twenty minutes, only feelings of confusion improved. After thirty minutes of sustained exercise, none of the negative moods saw further improvement.

Of course, exercising for longer has plenty of physical benefits, but the researchers concluded that exercising in short, ten-minute bursts a few times a day is enough to provide immediate improvements to your mood.

• *Schedule a short exercise break in the morning, afternoon, and evening to get the greatest emotional benefits from working out.*

Skip the Gym

You don't have to go to the fitness room to enjoy the emotional benefits of physical exercise. A group of German researchers examined how everyday physical activity affected three dimensions of mood: valence (its positivity or negativity), calmness, and energetic arousal. Using accelerometers, they tracked the physical activity of seventy-seven students during the relatively sedentary exam period, and had the students report their current moods hourly on a mobile app. Results showed that the more intense the activity (lasting for at least ten minutes), the more positive feelings increased. However, jogging for a half hour did not produce significantly different results than if the participants were just walking. The researchers suggested that breaking up an otherwise sedentary workday with daily activity like walking, stair climbing, or doing jumping jacks can improve your mood.

· *Even if you don't have time to get to the gym, take a break at work to walk a few blocks or climb a few flights of stairs to get into a better mood.*

WORKS BOTH WAYS

"It is generally assumed that physical exercise will add to your happiness, and correlational studies typically show a positive relation. Yet causality can work the other way–happiness stimulating physical exercise. . . . Feeling well makes people more active and outgoing."

–Ruut Veenhoven, professor emeritus of social conditions for human happiness, Erasmus University Rotterdam; founding director of the World Database of Happiness; a founding editor of the *Journal of Happiness Studies*

Feel Less Exhausted . . . by Working Out Longer

It may seem counterintuitive, but exercising longer can actually make you feel less exhausted.

Researchers looking at what effects gender, exercise type, exertion level, and length of workout had on mood recruited 135 participants and assigned them to either a weight training or cardiovascular exercise group. Participants were allowed to determine their own workout duration and exertion levels (the average length of their

SEVEN (MINUTES) TO SUCCEED

Taking these findings a step further, researchers at the Johnson & Johnson Human Performance Institute in Orlando, Florida, found that exercisers could reach "maximum results with minimal investment" through just seven minutes of high-intensity circuit training. Drawing on a range of physiological research going back decades, they determined that combining aerobic and resistance training in a series of exercises at high intensity, with limited rest, was a very effective way to trim fat and boost the heart rate.

To be most effective, the exercises should together work all muscles and each last long enough to get your heart racing, but without going so long that the intensity of the exercise decreases. Though the researchers found improvements with as little as four minutes total exercise time, the ideal balance to meet all these requirements is these twelve different exercises, performed for thirty seconds each with ten seconds rest between them:

1. Jumping jacks (total body)
2. Wall sit (lower body)
3. Push-up (upper body)
4. Abdominal crunch (core)
5. Step-up onto chair (total body)
6. Squat (lower body)
7. Triceps dip on chair (upper body)
8. Plank (core)
9. High knees/running in place (total body)
10. Lunge (lower body)
11. Push-up and rotation (upper body)
12. Side plank (core)

Squeeze in a seven-minute workout to ensure mood-boosting exercises are part of your daily routine.

workouts was 46.75 minutes, with a range between 10 and 120 minutes). Both before and after the test, they rated their levels of tension, depression, anger, vigor, and fatigue.

Results across the board showed higher mood ratings after exercising. But interestingly, the more difficult and longer the workout lasted, the more positive the mood participants reported. This was particularly true for weightlifting women, but generally true of all categories. Exhaustion ratings were also positively correlated with longer workout durations.

· If you consistently feel exhausted or less than positive after a workout, consider adding five more minutes to the next session.

Dehydration Can Be a Downer

We all know that we should drink more water. But beyond helping you feel better when you work out, hydration can actually help you perceive the effort involved in exercising as more manageable. Researchers tested twenty-five women on several cognitive tasks both while hydrated (after drinking 240 ml [about 8 ounces] of mineral water) and mildly dehydrated (after practicing moderate exercise).

While cognitive function itself was not reduced by dehydration, researchers found dehydration did increase subjects' perception of the task's difficulty, lowered their concentration and mood, and produced headache symptoms in those suffering only 1.36 percent dehydration levels.

· Drink water—even when you aren't thirsty.

Watch Out for Dry Eyes

Crying might usually seem a sign of sadness, but the truly sad people may be those with dry eyes. A team of ophthalmologists examined a group of 672 Japanese office workers, testing their dry-eye measurement using Schirmer's test (an assessment of whether an eye is producing enough tears to keep it moist) and their subjective happiness levels. Happiness was measured using the Subjective Happiness Scale, a survey developed by Sonja Lyubomirsky and Heidi S. Lepper in which respondents answer four questions, rating whether they consider themselves happy people on a scale from one (not very happy) to seven (very happy). The result was an inverse relationship between the two: Those with symptoms of dry eyes reported the lowest level of subjective happiness.

· *If your eyes are dry, get them checked out to avoid future tears.*

Get Older

Forget what you've heard about having a midlife crisis. In fact, getting older is a pretty good predictor of happiness. That was among the findings of a longitudinal study from the University of Alberta in Canada that looked at participants' happiness levels as they aged from eighteen to forty-three, with the participants self-defining and self-reporting their well-being on a scale from "not happy" to "very happy." The study found that over the twenty-five-year period, as individuals aged they generally grew happier. The increase in happiness remained even when controlling for variables like gender, marital status, unemployment, and physical health.

· *Stop worrying about getting older. Chances are that wherever you see yourself in five years, you're going to be happier when you get there.*

Filter Out the Negative

Additional research points to *why* older people tend to be happier: Younger adults focus on negative information more than positive information, while older adults put greater weight on positive memories and emotions. Those were the findings of a pair of studies conducted by a team of Stanford University researchers who asked subjects grouped by age to view positive, negative, and neutral images on a computer screen and then tested them for recognition and recall.

In the first study, the ratio of positive-to-negative material recalled increased with age—even as the older subjects' recall decreased overall. In the second study, the researchers used brain imaging to view how much the area processing emotion was activated as it viewed the different types of material. Older adults' brains activated much more for positive images than negative ones.

Drink More Coffee

If someone tells you they need coffee to survive, they might not be exaggerating. Spanish researchers following almost 20,000 people over a decade found that those who drank at least four cups per day had a 64 percent lower risk of dying—when researchers followed up about ten years after the initial assessment—than those who never or almost never consumed coffee. Though the researchers noted that this was just an observational study that could only make a correlation between the two, it does point to the possibility that caffeine is doing more than just keeping you awake.

· *Add an extra cup coffee or two to your daily routine.*

. . . Or Take a Break from Caffeine—Then Restart It

Caffeine has been shown to benefit alertness and cognitive functioning, but what effect does tolerance have on those benefits? It turns out a small increase in caffeine intake prior to completing a cognitive task boosts performance regardless of tolerance for caffeine.

This fact may also suggest that refraining from caffeine for short periods and then reestablishing consumption may lead to additional boosts.

These were the findings of a study conducted by researchers at the Wake Forest School of Medicine of seventeen people who consumed two to five cups of coffee per day, and who experienced withdrawal symptoms when they ceased using the caffeine. A baseline of caffeine consumption was established for each participant through a caffeine diary over seven consecutive days. Participants were then assigned to one of four groups: thirty-hour abstinence and placebo, thirty-hour abstinence and caffeine (250mg in capsule form), regular intake and placebo, or regular intake and caffeine (250mg in capsule form).

They then engaged in cognitive tasks and self-reported mood questionnaires. Caffeine was shown to have the greatest effect on mood after the subjects stopped drinking it for a period.

· *Improve your mood by cutting out coffee for a period and then start drinking it again.*

Eat Your Fruits and Vegetables

While we all know that eating more fruits and vegetables would be good for us, we don't usually think of them as happiness enhancers. As it turns out, bananas, broccoli, and other healthy foods can also improve one's well-being and life satisfaction. That was the finding of a study of 12,385 Australian adults' food diaries as logged in the Household, Income and Labour Dynamics in Australia Survey.

Researchers found a correlation between fruit and vegetable consumption and increased happiness and life satisfaction ratings. Furthermore, the changes were equal to the psychological gains of becoming employed if one was unemployed—though these mood-enhancing benefits were obtained after two years of dietary changes.

· *Changing your diet doesn't just create physical health benefits in the long term—it can also provide significant psychological benefits, too.*

SELECTIVELY OPTIMIZE

"Circumstances change as we move through the life course. A framework that I find useful is the theory [by Paul Baltes and Margaret Baltes] of selective optimization with compensation. The idea is that older people select and optimize their best abilities and most intact functions while compensating for declines and losses. However, I think the model can be applied to anyone who wants to take an active approach in setting work-life balance goals that are attainable and meaningful.

"As a dad of five children, I informally applied the SOC process even before it was proposed: I gave up golf and a number of other non-work passions while my children were growing up and cultivated other interests that I enjoyed (e.g., working with kids and coaching sports) that allowed me to share time with my children in fun and meaningful ways (for both them and me), and make a contribution to my community through volunteering. Having five children 'constrained me' into better achieving work-life balance as much as it always tried to evade my efforts."

–Roger C. Mannell

Grab Some Nuts

Fad diets come and go and promise all varieties of dubious life-changing benefits. But in the case of the Mediterranean diet (high in vegetables, fruits, and whole grains; low in red meat, butter, and processed foods), some science actually supports the assertion that it can boost a person's happiness—or at least reduce negative emotions—over the long term.

A team affiliated with Spain's Biomedical Research Networking Center for Physiopathology of Obesity and Nutrition assigned almost 4,000 participants to one of three groups: Mediterranean diet with extra virgin olive oil; Mediterranean diet with mixed nuts; or low-fat control group. The experimental groups were given intensive education on the Mediterranean diet and all participated in individual interviews and group sessions every three months, with a follow-up session once a year.

At the end of three years, 224 new cases of depression had been identified through diagnosis made by a physician or by the use of antidepressant medications. The researchers found an inverse relationship between depression and those eating the Mediterranean with nuts diet, which was especially pronounced when restricted to those with preexisting type 2 diabetes.

• *Add some more nuts and plants to your diet, and cut back on the red meat.*

Get Your Zs

Little can mess with your emotions more than a bad night—or several bad nights—of sleep. A wide range of studies have found that sleep difficulties are related to nearly all mood disorders, and the importance of adequate sleep has been observed clinically for many years. This is not just because being tired puts you in a bad mood. A literature review of the studies additionally found that the rapid eye movement (REM) stage of sleep is an integral part of emotional regulation in two ways: processing and synthesizing emotions from the previous day as memories are stored, and recalibrating emotion sensitivity for the next day. "Sleeping on it" actually creates enormous benefits for how you manage emotions.

· Rest is almost as important as exercise when it comes to your emotional well-being. Not feeling great? Give your emotions time to recharge.

Seven (Hours) to a Long Life

Daniel Kripke, codirector of research at the Scripps Clinic Sleep Center in San Diego, looked at the ultimate question when it comes to sleep and health: How long should you sleep to live a longer life? He examined data from 1.1 million men and women aged thirty to 102 and found that the best rate of survival was among those who slept about seven hours a night. Those sleeping less than six hours or more than eight hours experienced "significantly increased mortality hazard." This risk increased to more than 15 percent for those who slept less than 4.5 hours or more than 8.5 hours.

· Make seven hours your target amount of sleep. If you're way over or under, try going to bed at a different time, or changing your nighttime routines.

Skip the Sleeping Pills

Whatever you do to get your seven hours of sleep a night, medication is not a great long-term solution. The same sleep researcher found that long-term use of sleeping pills significantly increased one's risk of dying. So if you're having trouble sleeping, find ways to work through it beyond the pill bottle.

If You Miss Sleep, You Can Get It Back

A good night's sleep has been found to create a wide range of mental and physical health benefits. But if you toss and turn a few nights of the week, it turns out that catching up on the weekend can reverse the negative effects of the lost winks. A team of Korean researchers conducted in-person interviews with 2,156 adults about their sleep patterns, weight, mood, and other medical details. More than 900 of the subjects slept in on the weekend—what was technically called "catch-up sleep" or CUS—by an average of 0.7 to 2.9 hours more than on a typical weekday. Controlling for other factors, these late sleepers were found to have a lower body mass index than those who did not get the extra sleep.

• *Sleep in on the weekend, especially if you've had a few sleepless nights during the week.*

Work Out with Friends

Group physical activities can help improve exercise performance—and friendships. Those were the findings of a pair of studies from University of Oxford researchers who examined the performance of two groups of athletes. In the first study, they found that moderate-intensity exercise led to higher levels of cooperation in a game just afterward. In the second study, rugby players participated in solo, synchronized, and nonsynchronized warm-up sessions. Those who participated in the synchronized warm-up performed significantly better. So not only does group physical activity improve

EAT CHOCOLATE . . .
BUT BE MINDFUL ABOUT IT

Despite plenty of anecdotal evidence (and your weird aunt's many claims), there is little scientific support for the assertion that chocolate increases happiness. However, adding an extra ingredient into your chocolate consumption can turn it into a mood booster: mindfulness.

Researchers at Gettysburg College in Pennsylvania found that eating chocolate in a deliberate, slow way in which its color, taste, and tactile sensations were examined led to an increase in positive mood. They divided 258 participants into four groups and instructed each group to do one of the following:

❶ Mindfully consume crackers (intended as a control food)

❷ Mindfully consume chocolate

❸ Non-mindfully consume crackers

❹ Non-mindfully consume chocolate

While eating their assigned foods, participants followed audio-recorded directions (different for each group), and both before and after consuming their assigned foods, answered question-naires about their mood.

Those eating chocolate mindfully showed greater increases in positive mood than any of the other categories. Plus, a cor-relation was found between self-reported liking of the food and impact on mood ratings–in other words, those who liked choco-late experienced a greater boost of positive mood after mindful consumption.

· *Don't feel guilty about eating sweets–just be sure you are really thinking about them as you satisfy your sweet tooth.*

performance—it creates social bonding and leads to the formation of new relationships, both of which have been linked to happiness.

· *Recruit a buddy for your next workout.*

Competition Is More Motivating Than Encouragement

Another major advantage of being more social in exercising: competition. According to researchers at the University of Pennsylvania, friendly competition is the best source of motivation for those looking to exercise more. For the study, the researchers studied 790 members of the Penn community as they took part in an eleven-week exercise program that incorporated jogging, weight lifting, yoga, and more. Participants were randomly assigned to four different groups—individual competition, team competition, team support, and a control group—with members of each group receiving different types of messages and information via social networks. Those in the individual-competition group saw an exercise leaderboard that ranked the performance of each person in the group. Those in the team-support group could chat with each other, sending and receiving positive social media messages, but could not see the leaderboard. Those in the team-competition group could both exchange messages and see the leaderboard of rankings.

It turns out that competition makes a big difference. Both those in the team- and individual-competition groups attended far more workout sessions (an average of 38.5 and 35.7, respectively) than those in the control group (20.3 on average). But the team-support group members performed worse than everyone—attending just 16.8 workouts on average.

As the lead researcher, Damon Centola, put it, "Supportive groups can backfire because they draw attention to members who are less active, which can create a downward spiral of participation." Those who introduce a bit of competition between members "frame relationships in terms of goal-setting by the most active members. These relationships help to motivate exercise because they give people higher expectations for their own levels of performance."

• *Give your workouts a competitive edge by recruiting friends who will push you and whom you can push to do better.*

Track Your Food

Carefully monitoring what one eats is sometimes associated with an unhealthy obsession with dieting. But there's plenty of research that finds health benefits in tracking what you eat and when. A review of twenty-two studies published between 1993 and 2009, looking at the connection between self-monitoring of one's behavior and weight loss, found a consistent, positive association between the two.

The way that people tracked their diet, exercise, and weight—whether with a paper diary, electronic digital scale, mobile app, or otherwise—did not seem to matter. However, the researchers did suggest that the easier and faster the self-monitoring could be (e.g., access to an extensive database of foods that allows for fast entry of caloric information and ingredients), the more likely users would be to stick with it. The consistent result was that taking the extra time to think about what and how much they were eating, as well as their moods and the circumstances around when they ate, helped subjects to reevaluate their diets and gain greater awareness of their eating habits.

• *Take note of what you eat in a typical day, whether in a notepad or on your phone.*

. . . And Track Your Actions

Using an app or some other tool to track your healthy behaviors—and how they make you feel—can help to enhance your happiness. People have a tendency to suffer from recall bias—misremembering events or feelings that occurred in the past—so researchers sought to reduce this by asking subjects to log how healthy behaviors impacted their mood. In the study, 130 participants tracked their behaviors over a five-month period.

The results showed that people were in a better mood if they consumed more fruits and vegetables, weren't ill, got enough sleep, exercised longer, and traveled. People were generally in better moods during weekends. People were also in better moods if they had eaten fried food and drunk sugary drinks—though researchers were hesitant to endorse the positive effects of those unhealthy behaviors, suggesting that it may be eating in general that increased positive mood.

But what they could definitively conclude was that using an in-the-moment recall application or journaling style can help identify personal heath behavior patterns that contribute to your own happiness.

· *Track your healthy (or unhealthy) behavior to identify personal patterns that affect you throughout the day, as well as to increase your motivation to engage in more healthful behaviors once you've identified the effects they have on your overall happiness.*

Move–Right Now

Physical activity does not just have some vague long-term benefits. It causes immediate increases in one's level of happiness. That was a finding of a University of Cambridge study that took a step beyond retrospective self-reporting or reports for one specific period, to have more than 10,000 subjects report their happiness levels through a smartphone app.

Using the built-in accelerometer, the app could tell whether a person was active at the moment they reported their current mood. The results? Self-reported physical activity was positively related to happiness, as was physical activity sensed by the app. The research "reveals the important connection between physical and psychological processes, indicating that even slight changes in one has consequences for the other."

• *Stand up and run in place for a minute or do some stretches— movement boosts mood.*

The Cure for the Common Cold Might Be a Good Mood

Positive emotions can fight colds. A team of researchers exposed 193 participants to one of two strains of a cold (no, they didn't sneeze on them). Over a period of twenty-eight days, subjects recorded any symptoms they experienced, and their objective symptoms (mucus production, nasal clearance) were measured by the researchers. The subjects self-reported their own emotions throughout.

People who had more positive emotions (e.g., vigor, well-being, and calm) had lower reported symptoms, but not lower measured symptoms. But negative emotions (sadness, anxiety, and hostility) were not found to have a significantly negative impact on subjects' reported symptoms. It seems that positive emotions are more likely to help you fight a cold than negative emotions are to bring one on.

• *When trying to fight off a cold, add "think happy thoughts" to your regimen of vitamin C and cough syrup.*

Appreciate Your Body

While healthy activities improve one's mental health, thinking healthy does as well. Having a positive body image has been found to boost one's subjective level of happiness. A survey of 9,667 women about their body image found that those who expressed "body appreciation" were more likely to express higher levels of subjective happiness.

But while having a positive outlook on one's body created positive emotional benefits, body dissatisfaction actually had "no significant association with subjective happiness." The researchers concluded that instead of discouraging negative attitudes about one's body, greater improvements in one's emotional well-being are likely to come from focusing on the positive aspects of one's body, such as appreciating the body's functionality rather than its appearance.

• *Take a minute to appreciate how cool your body is—how much it can do and how effectively it is able to do it, from fingers to toes and everything in between.*

HiGh-Tech HaPPiNeSS

"True happiness is to enjoy the present, without anxious dependence upon the future, not to amuse ourselves with either hopes or fears but to rest satisfied with what we have, which is sufficient, for he that is so wants nothing."

–SENECA

Technology takes tremendous leaps every year and has made communicating with others faster, easier, and more efficient than ever. We can video chat, talk by phone, and send text messages in a matter of seconds. No wonder these devices have become a central part of our lives. A Gallup poll found that more than two fifths of adults check their smartphones multiple times *per hour*.

But as new technology is making some things easier, it is not making us happier. A quick review of the research that's been done about recent technology indicates that these hypnotic screens that have suddenly become so hugely important to modern life do exactly the opposite: Texting damages relationships, use of social media corrodes friendships, and the more you use the internet, the more likely you are to feel anxious—or worse.

But before you assume that this chapter is advocating unplugging from everything and moving to a cabin in the woods, read on.

While too much technology can eat away at well-being, there are many ways that using high-tech tools can make you feel better. From leveraging meditation and journaling apps to using Facebook to create the *right kind* of social capital, there are ways to use gadgets to better yourself. This chapter looks into what those are and how to make the machines work for you, rather than vice versa.

Ask: For What Are You Using the Internet?

It may not be the technology itself that impacts your happiness, but the ways you are using it. A look at internet usage and how it affects well-being found that the frequency of going online did not clearly correlate with well-being one way or another, but specific *types* of internet use correlated to depression, social anxiety, and family cohesion. The study isolated five main reasons individuals go online:

1. To meet people
2. To seek information
3. For distraction
4. To cope with a personal problem
5. To send/receive email

Those who went online for coping—using the internet to solve personal problems, try to "feel close to others," find information about topics they couldn't talk about with others, express themselves, and find distraction to relieve themselves from stress—were "more likely to report greater depression, greater social anxiety, and less family cohesion," according to the researchers. This contrasts with those who went online for more active tasks (such as seeking information or communicating with others) who reported higher levels of family cohesion—thanks, according to the researchers, to the day-to-day communication to loved ones it can provide.

• *If you use the internet to help you solve your personal problems, consider alternative, real-world ways to find these kinds of resources.*

Beware Internet Addiction

Another concern for frequent online users: internet addiction. The ping of an email hitting your inbox or a notification on Twitter releases a burst of dopamine much like what a smoker feels when lighting a cigarette. At one time or another, all of us have found ourselves opening a browser as soon as we wake up or surfing the web when we should have been doing something "better" with our time. But there's a big difference between that low-level wasting of time and full-on addiction.

A survey of 572 university students found that for at least 9 percent of those surveyed, the internet was an addiction, with these participants continuing to hop online even as they suffered adverse effects including exhaustion (after staying up late to browse) and academic problems. Those classified as addicts agreed that they shouldn't use the internet so much, as had been suggested to them by others, and thought that they would use it less if they had more friends. The researchers concluded that "the internet does play a role in some students' academic difficulties."

Stop Apologizing

If an email has been sitting in your inbox for a few days, or even a few hours, it often seems polite to begin your response by apologizing for your delayed response. Such anxiety about responding immediately might make you think you are being conscientious, but in fact you are just driving yourself crazy. One study found that people respond to emails, on average, within six seconds. Yet in almost all cases, the sender does not actually expect an immediate response. Duke University psychology professor Dan Ariely conducted a test, asking people who emailed him to fill out a form and indicate if they required an answer right away. Just 2 percent actually needed an immediate answer.

· Remove "Apologies for the delay" from your email vocabulary. There is a high likelihood the recipient didn't even notice.

Dunbar's Number Works on Twitter

You may have thousands of followers on Twitter, but how many of them do you actually know? Dunbar's number—the approximate number of people in your social circle with whom you can maintain a meaningful relationship (discussed in Chapter 6)—has also been found to apply to social media. A team of researchers from Indiana University analyzed data of Twitter conversations collected over a six-month period to test whether this concept—developed before the invention of microblogging—might still apply. Analyzing more than 380 million tweets involving 1.7 million individuals, they determined that users were able to maintain a maximum of one hundred to two hundred stable social media relationships over time.

· Don't expect your tweets to appeal to all your followers all the time; just focus on your 150 closest friends.

Turn Off Your Social Networks

While social networks are where we go to keep in touch with friends, acquaintances, and people with whom we might not otherwise correspond, they may actually be hurting our social life. Researchers at Florida State University and Florida International University looking at factors that mitigate stress and boost life satisfaction in college students found social networking and texting to be correlated with both lower levels of life satisfaction and higher levels of stress.

As the researchers put it, texting and social media "allow the user to disengage from the demands of real-time social interaction" that would be required in a phone call or face-to-face conversation. The finding that heavy social media users are also less likely to be in a romantic relationship is a bit ironic, considering that many students use social networking cites to find dates. But the research suggests that these behaviors lead to isolation and depression symptoms.

· *Instead of "Liking" someone's status on Facebook, message them to see if they want to grab a drink.*

Don't Trust Apps to Find You Love

Speaking of technology and dating: Tinder may have plenty of users, but apps are not reliable tools for finding love, according to researchers. A study by a team of psychologists tested how skilled sophisticated machine learning was at predicting individuals' romantic desire for one another—and the machines failed. The researchers asked participants to answer more than one hundred questions about personality traits and preferences in romantic partners. The researchers next used an advanced algorithm to predict which other participants each would be attracted to, based on their corresponding responses. Subjects then took part in four-minute speed dates, noting their level of interest in each person they met.

The algorithm failed to identify any pattern in the participants' answers sufficient to predict whether any two subjects would be likely to connect. As the study's authors put it, "compatibility elements of human mating are challenging to predict before two people meet."

· *Apps can't predict whether you will hit it off with someone; your odds of success are much higher if you simply approach a person in person.*

Take a Social Sabbatical

A team of Danish researchers asked a group of almost 1,100 subjects to stop using Facebook for one week. The participants were asked before and after the break to rate, on a scale of one (very dissatisfied) to ten (very satisfied), "How satisfied are you with your life today?"

Those in the control group remained at about the same average, while those who quit Facebook for a week went from an average of 7.56 to an average of 8.12. The Facebook quitters also described feeling a big increase in their concentration, decisiveness, enthusiasm, and more.

· *Take a break from your newsfeed. Even if it's just for a few days, it can have a big impact.*

REFRAME YOUR SMARTPHONE RELATIONSHIP

"I never hear people tell me in clinical practice that people hope that their family and friends will remember them for the time they spent at work or on their smartphones—and yet, this is where we seem to be spending more and more of our days. While this time is spent under the pretext of being 'productive,' often it is more about seeking pleasure and avoiding discomfort. Smartphones are like slot machines, designed to grab your attention and reward the brain and body with short hits of pleasure—unless you are aware of this and can use them wisely and with intention.

"Reflect on and consider the type of relationship that you want with your phone, just as you should any relationship in your life. Get intentional about it. Consider the function of the ways you interact with your phone. Is it about distraction and avoidance or is it about the things that we know lift our spirits and create pathways to connection, meaning, and happiness in our lives?"

–Jo Mitchell, clinical psychologist

Text for "Relationship Maintenance"

As anyone who has sent a random kissy-face emoji knows, texting can have a healthy place in relationships. Researchers at Brigham Young University looked at the texting behavior of 276 young adults from around the United States to examine how it impacted their relationships. They found that texting to express affection was associated with higher levels of attachment between the partners, but other kinds of texting were associated with lower relationship quality:

For men, it was found that overly frequent texting might be taking a toll on their relationships.

For women, it has been found that using text messages to apologize, make decisions, or work out differences may in fact be causing distance.

· *Stick with flirty and affectionate subjects in your texts to a partner; anything more serious is probably better handled in person.*

Talk, Don't Text, Over Long Distances

Modern technology would seem to hold an ideal solution for a relatively old-fashioned challenge, the long-distance relationship. The other person can seem so far away, making communication more important than ever in order to maintain a sense of connection. But in a study of how different types of communication impacted satisfaction with relationships, some methods clearly had advantages over others.

The study looked at 311 unmarried participants who were separated from their partners by distances ranging from ninety miles to more than 10,000 miles, for periods ranging from about two weeks to more than ten years. Those who used webcams and phone calls—methods most similar to face-to-face communication—were more likely to express feeling emotionally supported by their partner and social with their partner, and that they were the recipient of advice and guidance.

On the other hand, there was no positive correlation found between text messaging or instant messaging and respondents' feelings of emotional support, advice or guidance, or socializing. Alarmingly, frequency of text messaging (which has become a go-to means of communicating for many people) was actually found to be negatively correlated with relationship satisfaction; the more partners communicated by text, the less happy they were.

This study indicates that more intimate forms of communication (face to face, telephone calls, and letter writing) remain the most effective communication methods when it comes to keeping love alive over great distances.

· *Use Skype or Facetime to keep your long-distance relationship going long term.*

Texting Kills Your GPA

On the list of negative side effects of excessive texting, you can add that it hurts your grades. A study that examined the relationship between cell phone usage/texting and life satisfaction of a group of 500 college students found cell phone use and texting was negatively correlated to subjects' grade point averages. The students surveyed spent a jaw-dropping average of 278.67 minutes (almost 4-¾ hours) per day on their cell phones and sent an average of 76.68 text messages.

It turned out that high-frequency cell phone users tended to have lower GPAs and lower life satisfaction relative to their peers who used their phones less often. The researchers suggested this might be due to the fact that those using cell phones a lot are not focusing on academic work, or are using them during class or when they should be studying. As they put it, "In other words, high frequency

ELEVATE YOUR PHONE USAGE

Technology is not always bad, of course. Anyone who has turned to their smartphone when lost in the middle of a city or to watch a cat video when they really needed a pick-me-up knows that having a high-tech device on hand has its perks. That's why Jo Mitchell, clinical psychologist and director of The Mind Room, a well-being center based in Melbourne, Australia, urges finding ways to elevate your smartphone usage, to turn it into a source of fulfillment instead of depletion. There are three key ways you can do this:

❶ **Connection:** Facebook and social media can offer big social benefits, if used properly. "We know that the strongest predictor of happiness in life is the quality of our social connections, so anything we do to nurture those and to feel valued and appreciated by others is great for our health and well-being, and for theirs," as Mitchell puts it.

❷ **Mindfulness:** Using mindfulness apps such as Buddhify, Headspace, or Smiling Mind can turn your phone into an oasis of calm. "Suddenly meditation practice is not location bound–it can travel with you wherever you are and fit in the gaps of your life," she says. "In an attention economy, learning to be master of your own mind, rather than slave to it, is key to happiness."

❸ **Charity:** Selfless acts and charity have been found to boost one's well-being significantly. Your mobile device can help you to do that more effectively. "Send a Touchnote postcard to a friend via your phone to their real-world postbox (remember them?)," says Mitchell. "Or donate to a cause using apps like Shout for Good."

users are more likely to be multitasking and task switching while in class or studying and these behaviors are known to lower academic performance."

· Each ping may distract you from the task at hand, so try silencing your phone altogether or keeping it out of sight to improve your overall performance—in class or otherwise.

Cell Phones Increase Anxiety

The same study found that that while high cell phone usage hurt GPAs, it also ratcheted up anxiety. The researchers theorized that this may be due to the fact that the ever-present mobile device makes it difficult for users to disconnect and "find the solitude necessary to temporarily escape these perceived obligations"—an important component of well-being and life satisfaction.

· Turn off your notifications—or turn off your mobile device altogether— for designated periods of time throughout the day in order to allow yourself breaks to be present in the moment.

Keep It Personal

If you want to help increase the happiness of your friends, stop "Liking" them. A study from Carnegie Mellon University looked at more than 1,900 Facebook users' activity logs over three months and how they corresponded with their self-reports of psychological well-being. While comments with a personal touch corresponded with improved happiness, "Likes" and similar one-click communications made no improvement in the subjects' well-being.

· Next time you're about to click that "Like" button for a friend's post, think of something more personal to say and write it in the comment field—or say it to them in person.

USE FACEBOOK TO BUILD OFFLINE SOCIAL CAPITAL

As this chapter has so far demonstrated, social media is often a weak stand-in for actual in-person socializing. But it does have some real-world advantages. A team of researchers from Michigan State University surveyed 286 undergraduate students and found Facebook usage to be positively associated with three types of social benefits:

❶ **Bridging social capital:** connections to people from different walks of life than your own—weaker ties than you might have with close friends, but ones that enable social inclusion to a wider variety of groups

❷ **Bonding social capital:** connections to like-minded people— family, team or organization members, or hometown friends

❸ **Maintained social capital:** relationships you continue even after relocating or changing jobs or interests

A positive relationship was found between Facebook use and the building and maintenance of all three of these types of connections. Interestingly, general internet use didn't help build capital, except in the case of maintained social capital. Students reporting low life satisfaction and low self-esteem gained bridging social capital when they used Facebook more heavily. The researchers pointed out that using social media does not remove one from the real world, but "may indeed be used to support relationships and keep people in contact, even when life changes move them away from each other."

Stop Comparing, Start Appreciating

One of the biggest reasons Facebook and Twitter negatively impact happiness is the social comparisons that you are likely to make when scrolling through your newsfeed. You may be feeling pretty good with how your day is going only to see that a friend is relaxing on some Caribbean beach or just got a big promotion at work. Or you just bought a new bike you're excited about—and a high school buddy posts a photo of her fancy new car. The fact that such "upward comparisons" push our mood downward has been established through studies going back to at least the 1950s.

While it's hard to avoid doing this, Mai-Ly Steers of the University of Houston suggested to James Hamblin of the *Atlantic* that "the antidote to comparison tends to be gratitude. If you're grateful for things, you're not really comparing yourself."

· *If an acquaintance's boastful post has you feeling down, think of something that's good in your life. You could even express gratitude for the fact that you have successful acquaintances. If that fails to dislodge your depression, get off Facebook and go do something that makes you proud.*

Play More Video Games

While spending your life with an Xbox controller in hand is not the most fulfilling way to live, there may be some benefits to gaming—particularly for the elderly. A team of researchers from Singapore's Nanyang Technological University found that Wii-type games allow the elderly to socialize and exercise while playing. They studied a group of forty-five residents of a senior home and found that the games improve functional abilities like hand-eye coordination and balance, which in turn reduce the incidence of falls among the elderly.

In addition to the physical benefits, the study found that "seniors who played Wii are better off in their psychological well-being than seniors who engaged in traditional activities." They scored significantly higher on self-esteem and affect, and significantly lower on loneliness, compared to those in the control group. Of course, the findings were limited to older folks and to active games that involved physical motion—sitting on the couch playing the latest *Resident Evil* probably would not generate the same positive results.

Snap a Selfie

While endlessly photographing yourself is a bit narcissistic, it has been found to be an effective way to give yourself a jolt of joy. Researchers at the University of California, Irvine's Donald Bren School of Information and Computer Sciences assigned forty-one college students to three different groups. The first was instructed to take a smiling selfie each day; the second was told to take an image of something that made them happy; and the third to take a picture of something they thought would bring happiness to another person and then send the image to others.

Over a period of four weeks, the researchers collected almost 2,900 measurements of the subjects' moods, and found that those in all three categories experienced upticks in their happiness levels. Their reasons for this varied: selfie takers reported that their smile became more natural over time, while those taking photos of the things that made them happy said they became more appreciative of the little things that brought them joy in life. Those taking pictures and sending them to others reported feeling more connected to the people to whom they sent the photos and felt a reduction in stress.

· *Turn your cell phone camera into a happiness booster by snapping a smiling pic of yourself or something you like once a day. That doesn't mean you have to share those selfies on Instagram—at least not every day.*

More Radio and Less TV

Old-school media can influence your well-being in important ways. The effects of watching TV are very different from listening to the radio or reading a newspaper. In the United States, people spend around five hours per day watching TV; in Europe, around three hours. Both would probably do well to cut down.

In Europe, people who watch more than half an hour of TV a day report that they are less satisfied with their lives than those who watch less or none. No such result was reported for listening to the radio. In fact, listening to the radio for more than two hours a day makes people happier than not listening at all.

Reading newspapers has been found to have a similar, and even greater, positive effect to people's happiness as listening to the radio. Those who read newspapers are much happier than those who do not, and the more time they spend with newspapers, the happier they are.

· Listen to a podcast or the radio for thirty minutes more than you usually do, and watch TV for thirty minutes less.

. . . Though Watching TV with a Significant Other Can Be Healthy

Too much television is not generally good for your happiness level—unless you watch it with a spouse or significant other. Shared media experiences—reading the same books, sharing a movie night together, or watching the same TV shows—have been found to create stronger connections in couples. Researchers conducted a pair of studies and found that while sharing real social worlds (i.e., having living, breathing mutual friends) predicted a greater quality of relationships in couples, in cases where members of a couple lacked mutual friends, a shared media world could promote a better relationship between the two.

• *Netflix and chill with your significant other—unless you have real friends to hang out with.*

9

FiNDiNG YOUR HaPPY PLaCE

"It is impossible for a man to be made happy, by putting him into a happy place; unless he be first in a happy state."

–BENJAMIN WHICHCOTE

So far, we've focused mostly on what makes a person happy, but here we briefly broaden things out. What makes a city happy? Or a country? Urban planners, economists, psychologists, and many others have looked into these questions over decades, finding a wide range of variables that shape the general well-being of a population. Of course, it's difficult to precisely say what makes a perfect place for widespread happiness, considering the wide range of preferences and motivators that drive those who live there or might want to move there. Quality healthcare and a pleasant climate might be priorities for elderly citizens, but a great nightlife and plenty of job opportunities are the more likely attractions for twentysomethings. Drawing on socioeconomic, demographic, and geographic data along with population-wide surveys and more, researchers have been able to isolate certain things that make a place more appealing, livable, and conducive to generating happiness in the population at large.

Here we look at what researchers have determined to be the happiest countries in the world, and what it takes to become a place of widespread happiness—what makes a happy place, and how you can go about finding it.

Get Out of Town

It's become almost a cliché that big cities can wear down your happiness and that moving out to a quieter place more deeply connected with nature can improve your mood. But there is evidence to support this. The General Social Survey (GSS), conducted by the National Opinion Research Center at the University of Chicago since 1972, gathers Americans' demographic and behavioral information as well as their attitudes on a range of topics, such as stress, social mobility, and spending habits. Drawing on data from the GSS from 1972 to 2008, public policy researchers at the University of Texas at Dallas found that people in major cities do indeed express lower levels of subjective well-being than those in small towns or rural areas.

The data shows that people living in small towns and rural areas generally report being happier, even when controlling for other variables—likely driven, according to the researchers, by the lower density and greater homogeneity in these more low-key areas.

. . . Or Do Cities Get a Bad Rap?

Harvard economics professor Edward Glaeser begs to differ. In his book *Triumph of the City*, he makes the case that cities are "our species' greatest invention." He counters the reports of how urban centers can wear on citizens' happiness with data that demonstrates the opposite: 30 percent of those living in countries where more than half the population is urban say they are very happy, compared to 25 percent who say the same in countries where more than half the population is rural. On the other end, just 17 percent of citizens in majority urban countries say they are not very or not at all happy, compared with 22 percent of those in majority rural countries.

He points out that "[a]cross countries, reported life satisfaction rises with the share of the population that lives in cities, even when controlling for the countries' income and education."

Measuring Quality of Life

Researchers have been gauging the "goodness of life" in US cities at least as far back as the 1930s. But the first comprehensive approach, based on statistical evidence, to measuring the quality of life on a citywide and regional level seems to have been by David Smith, in his book *The Geography of Social Well-Being*. The book, published in 1974, looked at statistical data for poverty, health care delivery, environmental quality, and other factors believed to have an effect on well-being. However, at least one critic at the time commented that the variables he chose to determine these happy places (e.g., welfare payments, diets, incomes) were "somewhat arbitrary, largely a function of what is publicly available. . . . Venereal disease is given as much weight as poverty."

But early efforts to determine the happiest cities evolved, with researchers looking at the type of amenities in a given city, as well as using more sophisticated measurement of variables to work out more objective quality-of-life scores for cities, states, and countries.

SEEK SOCIAL SUPPORT AND ECONOMIC STABILITY

The *World Happiness Report*, from the United Nations' Sustainable Development Solutions Network, bases its ranking on a simple number: the average answer of how the citizens of each country evaluate the quality of their lives, on a scale from zero to ten. Specifically, respondents are asked this question, based on the research of Hadley Cantril: "Imagine a ladder, with steps numbered from 0 at the bottom to 10 at the top. The top of the ladder represents the best possible life for you and the bottom of the ladder represents the worst possible life for you. On which step of the ladder would you say you personally feel you stand at this time?"

According to the *World Happiness Report*, these were the countries where citizens felt highest on the ladder–and the top performers have changed little since the first report in 2012:

	2017	2012
1	Norway	Denmark
2	Denmark	Finland
3	Iceland	Norway
4	Switzerland	The Netherlands
5	Finland	Canada
6	The Netherlands	Switzerland
7	Canada	Sweden
8	New Zealand	New Zealand
9	Australia	Australia
10	Sweden	Ireland

Three quarters of the differences among countries, and also among regions, are accounted for by differences in six key variables, according to the UN:

1. GDP per capita

2. Healthy years of life expectancy

3. Social support (as measured by having someone to count on in times of trouble)

4. Trust/absence of corruption (as measured by a perceived absence of corruption in government and business)

5. Freedom to make life decisions

6. Generosity (as measured by one's most recent three donations)

GIVE EUROPE A LOOK

The consulting firm Mercer has developed its own quality of living rankings aimed at identifying the places in the world that are safest and most desirable to live. This information is then used by companies to help decide where to set up offices or send workers. Mercer assesses living conditions based on thirty-nine factors, which it groups into ten categories:

1. Political and social environment (political stability, crime, law enforcement)

2. Economic environment (currency exchange regulations, banking services)

3. Sociocultural environment (media availability and censorship, limitations on personal freedom)

④ Medical and health considerations (medical supplies and services, infectious diseases, sewage, waste disposal, air pollution)

⑤ Schools and education (standards and availability of international schools)

⑥ Public services and transportation (electricity, water, public transportation, traffic congestion)

⑦ Recreation (restaurants, theaters, cinemas, sports and leisure)

⑧ Consumer goods (availability of food and daily consumption items, cars)

⑨ Housing (rental housing, household appliances, furniture, maintenance services)

⑩ Natural environment (climate, record of natural disasters)

Drawing on these factors, here are the top ten cities to live in for 2017:

① Vienna, Austria

② Zurich, Switzerland

③ Auckland, New Zealand

④ Vancouver, Canada

⑤ Dusseldorf, Germany

⑥ Frankfurt, Germany

⑦ Geneva, Switzerland

⑧ Copenhagen, Denmark

⑨ Basel, Switzerland

⑩ Sydney, Australia

Equality Benefits All

A team of psychologists drawing on General Social Survey data found that Americans were on average happier in the years when income inequality was lower. They found this was due to the fact that in years with greater disparity between income levels, there were higher levels of perceived unfairness and lower levels of trust. When there was more national income inequality, Americans trusted each other less.

Perhaps unsurprisingly, the negative association between income disparity and happiness could be seen in those respondents with lower incomes, but not those who had higher incomes. But it was not the reduced income that was found to dampen the low-income respondents' happiness—it was their lower level of perceived trust. The researchers conclude that "income growth without income disparity is likely to result in an increase in the mean happiness of a general population."

Epidemiologists Richard Wilkinson and Kate Pickett extended this argument even further: They found evidence that a wide range of problems are worse in places with greater inequality—regardless of how rich or poor the places are. This was the case in all fifty states in the US, as well as twenty-three of the richest countries in the world. Among the problems that are exacerbated when the gap between rich and poor grows: drug abuse, teen pregnancy, violence, obesity, and imprisonment rates. And among the things that are negatively impacted by inequality: physical health, mental health, child well-being, social mobility, and, of course, trust.

Inequality Index

Economist Wim Kalmijn and happiness studies pioneer Ruut Veenhoven, both of Erasmus University Rotterdam, have come up with an index of inequality-adjusted happiness, which doesn't just look at the average level of happiness in a country, but also at the relative inequality between citizens. Of the fifteen nations reviewed in their study, Denmark topped the list, with a score of seventy-five out of one hundred. Tanzania was at the bottom, with just twenty-two.

Emotion Matters

Individualist nations can be very emotional. In a comparison of life satisfaction of sixty-one nations, researchers at the University of Illinois at Urbana-Champaign found different predictors of life satisfaction in countries considered individualist (those emphasizing personal achievement, self-reliance, and competition, such as the United States and those in Western Europe) versus collectivist (those emphasizing cohesion, unity, and family and work organizations, such as China or Korea).

Looking at responses from more than 62,000 people, the researchers found that in individualist cultures, emotions were significant predictors of life satisfaction. In collectivist nations, normative beliefs were equally as strong as emotions in predicting life satisfaction—for example, the sense that a person is living up to their role as a spouse or employee. The researchers determined that while 40 percent of the variance in life satisfaction of those in collectivist nations could be attributed to norms, that was true for just 12 percent of the variation in individualist nations.

On the other hand, while 39 percent of the variance in collectivist nations was due to emotions, almost double that—76 percent— shaped life satisfaction in individualist nations. The findings pointed to the fact that, as the researchers put it, "regardless of why or how a person feels a specific emotion," the way it actually influences their life depends on their culture.

Consider the Ideal Affect

Rather than examining how someone actually feels (i.e., whether they are happy or sad), some researchers now also consider how subjects *prefer* to feel. Stanford University associate professor of psychology Jeanne Tsai defines this as the "ideal affect." She illustrates it with a comparison between North Americans (who in surveys expressed a preference for "high arousal affect" such as excitement and enthusiasm), and East Asians (who prefer "low arousal affect" such as calm and peacefulness). As she puts it, "people do different things to feel good because they differ in their ideal affect."

PURSUING A DIFFERENT HAPPINESS

"After a decade of research, Jeanne Tsai's propositions about ideal affect have largely been supported. Having said this, it's important to remember that these are cultural tendencies. North Americans, too, want to experience low arousal affect at certain times and for certain reasons and so engage in more passive leisure activities. Similarly, Chinese, too, want to experience high arousal affect at certain times and for certain reasons and so engage in more active leisure activities.

"So, the benefits accrued from engaging in leisure are similar in nature (e.g., wanting to decrease the discrepancy between ideal and actual affect), but different in kind (e.g., wanting to do so in terms of high arousal affect versus low arousal affect), across cultures."

–Gordon J. Walker, professor of kinesiology, sport, and recreation,
University of Alberta

Freedom Beats Money

Just as money can't buy you happiness as an individual, that may also be the case as a nation. Nobel Prize–winning economist Amartya Sen has found that in places experiencing an expansion of relative freedom, economic growth and quality of life have followed. He suggests that countries would be better off by focusing on expanding freedom—ensuring that people are able to live the way they want to as much as possible—rather than on income levels or gross national product. As he puts it, "An alternative to focusing on means of good living is to concentrate on the *actual living* that people manage to achieve."

Host a Sports Event

It's not whether you win or lose, it's if you host the game. A study of twelve European countries found that hosting an international sporting event—the Olympics, FIFA World Cup, or Union of European Football Associations (UEFA) European Championship—gave a significant boost to self-reports of life satisfaction among their populations. The "feel-good factor" a person enjoys from having their country host a sports event is as large as the increase in satisfaction one derives from getting married—if not as long lasting.

However, the researchers found no significant relation between national happiness and success or "[b]etter than expected national athletic performance in the national game"—for example, one's country winning more Olympic medals than expected. Turns out, just being a generous host is enough to boost the national mood.

A Surprising Statistic

In examining happy places, economists from the University of Warwick in England, Hamilton College (Clinton, NY), and the Federal Reserve Bank of San Francisco came upon a troubling finding: The happiest places on earth often have the highest suicide rates. Drawing on life satisfaction scores for US states, subjective well-being rankings from the World Values Survey, and suicide rates, the researchers found a consistent correlation between happy places and high suicide rates.

The researchers suggested that the reason for this is not that happier people are more prone to taking their own lives, but that "although one's own happiness protects one from suicide ... the level of others' happiness is a risk factor." They pointed to a number of studies looking at other areas of life—unemployment, obesity, crime—that find that individuals judge themselves less harshly when other people have outcomes similar to theirs. However, if you are feeling unhappy and those around you feel pretty cheery, it may only deepen your depression.

This dark side to happiness makes for a fitting transition to the next chapter, which looks at the less pleasant aspects of the pursuit of happiness.

10

The DOWNSiDe OF HaPPiNeSS

"Sanity and happiness are an impossible combination."

–MARK TWAIN, *THE MYSTERIOUS STRANGER*

Maybe it's a little late to bring this up, but being happy is not always a good thing. This book has largely come from the position that happiness is a desirable state of being and that becoming happy will enhance your work, life, and relationships. While that's largely true, there are also times when happiness can be a problem, or *ways* of being happy that can create issues in your life—or even end it altogether. It turns out that happiness is not the answer to everything.

This chapter looks at when happiness can be trouble, or at least it makes the case that having a smile on your face will not solve all of your problems. Here are tips about when tempering your emotions can be advantageous, and ways to leverage negativity, which will have a positive impact on your life satisfaction over the long term. Whether it's spotting liars, getting more creative, or simply avoiding turning into a psychopath, here is how a cloudier disposition can work to your benefit.

There's More to Life Than Happiness

Happiness gets a lot of attention, but researchers believe that looking beyond just that one big, shiny emotion is actually necessary to achieve greater emotional health. Those examining these questions have found benefits in thinking of emotional health not as a simple sliding scale of happy to miserable, but as something like an emotional ecosystem where a balance of different emotions or "emodiversity" (amusement, joy, awe, contentment, gratitude, etc.) results in greater health than a simple positive disposition. A team of researchers conducted a pair of cross-sectional studies of more than 37,000 respondents and found that high levels of emodiversity (measured in ways similar to how natural sciences quantify the biodiversity of ecosystems) were associated with better mental and physical health than was a high concentration of a specific positive emotion and not others.

This can affect physical health as well. A professor of human development and gerontology drew on diary data from 175 adults who tracked their positive and negative emotions at the end of each day over a thirty-day period. Those who had greater diversity in their positive emotions were found to be healthier; specifically, they had lower levels of inflammatory activity that can contribute to type 2 diabetes, rheumatoid disease, and more.

· *Embrace a range of positive emotions, thinking of happiness as one useful mood among many.*

Mixed Emotions Boast Benefits

A pair of psychologists studied mixed emotional experience and its impact on psychological well-being, monitoring a group of forty-seven subjects over twelve weekly therapy sessions. They found that the experience of happiness and sadness at the same time was a consistent precursor to significant psychological self-improvement over time. "Thus, while the concurrent experience of happiness and sadness in the face of adversity might not provide immediate benefit, it may signal enhancements in psychological well-being in the near future," wrote the authors.

· *Embrace wins* and *losses. Taking them together will position you for longer-term improvements.*

Pursuing Happiness Can Make You Sad

More concerning, it turns out that trying to increase your level of happiness can lead to the exact opposite. It seems that the greater value you put on happiness, the more likely you are to feel disappointed in failing to achieve it. One study asked subjects to "try to make yourself feel as happy as possible," while they listened to a piece of music. Those urged to put themselves in a positive mood reported feeling less happy than those who were given no instructions.

In another study, the more subjects reported valuing happiness, the less psychological well-being and life satisfaction they expressed, as well as greater mental health challenges such as depression. In a separate study, subjects read a fake news article that either described the benefits of happiness or did not mention it. Participants then watched a happy or sad film clip. Those who were prompted to value happiness reported feeling worse after watching the happy film than those who did not receive the prompt.

Pursuing Happiness Can Hurt Your Relationships

Working too hard to be happy can also negatively impact your relations with others. In one study, the more the subjects expressed valuing happiness, the lonelier they expressed feeling in daily diary entries. In another, those who were induced to place a greater value on happiness ended up feeling a greater sense of social disconnection. Researchers examining these patterns suggested that one of the reasons for this pattern is that pursuing happiness for personal gain alienates others.

So does that mean you need to give up being happy in order to *be* happy? Not quite. It turns out that just as desiring positive feelings you don't experience can make you feel worse, the reverse is also true: Accepting negative feelings can help you get past them quicker than those who fight against them. For example, a study gave one of three instructions (accept, suppress, or control) to subjects suffering from a panic disorder. Those who were instructed to feel acceptance felt less anxiety than the other two groups during a test that could trigger panic.

· *Accept negative feelings as a natural part of daily life. You can't be happy all the time.*

Too Much Happiness Makes You . . .

Happiness has so many benefits in one's life, it might seem like the more you have, the better off you are. But there is such a thing as too much happiness. A pair of researchers used Aristotle's idea of "moderation in all things" to suggest that positive traits "reach inflection points at which their effects turn negative"—for example, too much generosity leads to wastefulness, too much courage to recklessness.

This is known in psychology as an "inverted U," where the best performance occurs when there are moderate levels of a good thing, then drops precipitously when levels move too far in the direction of a deficiency or an excess on either side. A similar idea can be applied to happiness itself. When your level of happiness gets dangerously high, it can lead to a number of negative results.

. . . Take Too Many Risks

Psychologists have found that reaching constant high levels of happiness can lead to risky behavior as you seek out the next happiness high. This could include thrill seeking through drug use, or the perpetual hunt for novelty—not just in experiences, but in one's partners, spouses, and other areas that are best kept constant. Psychologists maintain that this can create instability in a person's life, resulting in unhappiness over the long term.

Researchers looking into this question found that those experiencing heightened emotional states (both positive and negative) were more likely to engage in rash actions such as high alcohol consumption, risky sexual behavior, and binge eating.

One study even found a high degree of "cheerfulness/optimism" in children, as rated by their parents and teachers, to be associated with a shorter life. Using a sample of more than 1,200 California students tracked over seven decades, the study found that high levels of cheerfulness were associated with a reduced lifespan. Specifically, those in the 75th percentile on cheerfulness had 123 percent of the risk of dying in a given year, compared to a person in the 25th percentile of cheerfulness (by comparison, high cholesterol is associated with a 120 percent risk). In contrast, a higher rating of conscientiousness predicted a longer life—someone with a high level of prudence and truthfulness had 77 percent of the risk of dying in a given year compared to a person with a lower level of conscientiousness.

. . . Worse at Spotting Liars

A study from the University of New South Wales in Australia found that happier people are also more gullible. Participants watched a ten-minute video aimed at generating either positive, negative, or neutral feelings (clips of a British comedy series for positive; an excerpt from a film about dying of cancer for negative; a nature documentary for neutral). They then viewed four brief interrogation videos of men and women denying that they'd committed a theft: University students in the videos entered a room in which there was a movie ticket in an envelope; they could either take the ticket or leave it, but either way had to deny taking it.

The participants watched videos in which some students truthfully denied having taken the ticket, while others lied. Those who watched the happy or sad videos were about equally effective in identifying students telling the truth. But those who watched the sad video before the interrogation videos proved much better at ferreting out the liars. So anyone considering working as a fraud investigator or judge might want to seek out a few tearjerkers on Netflix.

. . . Less Accurate

Researchers have developed the concept of "depressive realism"—that depressed people have a more accurate view of the world around them and their place in it. In a series of experiments, psychologists Lauren B. Alloy and Lyn Y. Abramson tapped 144 depressed and 144 nondepressed students to look at this effect. Participants were asked to press a button; a green light then would or would not turn on. In reality, they had no control over the light since the researchers were dictating whether or not to turn the light on. When asked to rate the level of control they felt they had over the light, the nondepressed subjects overestimated how much control they had, while the depressed students were much more accurate.

Similar results have been found in a number of other studies in which subjects were asked to make self-assessments, with depressed individuals proving more accurate. So what one person considers pessimistic may indeed just be realistic.

. . . More Rigid

According to psychologists Barbara Fredrickson and Marcial Losada, the ideal balance of positive emotions to negative emotions during the day may be about three to one (more precisely, 2.9 to one). They drew this number from a study in which a group of 188 people made daily reports for about a month, documenting when they experienced positive and negative emotions. Those whose positive emotions outweighed negative ones by a mean ratio of 2.9 or a little more were found to be "flourishing"—what the researchers defined as operating at an optimal level of functioning and health. Those who dipped below that line, whether as individuals, marriage partners, or members of business teams, tended to "languish."

But if the ratio goes too far in the positive direction, it can lead to people getting stuck in their ways. According to Fredrickson and Losada, people with extremely high positive-to-negative-emotion ratios (of more than five to one or so) have been found to be more rigid in their behavior. As they put it, "Without appropriate negativity, behavior patterns calcify."

. . . Less Creative

In a meta-analysis of the relationship between mood and creativity, the University of North Texas's Mark A. Davis found that moderate levels of positivity can help open up our minds and get us to think outside the box. But those experiencing *high* levels of happiness did not exhibit the same burst of creativity as those feeling moderately cheery.

. . . Psychopathic?

An extreme level of heightened positive emotion and lack of negative emotion may be an indicator of psychopathology, or at least abnormality. In 1992, University of Liverpool professor Richard Bentall laid out the case for classifying happiness as a psychiatric disorder. He concluded that it does indeed meet most criteria for this: "Happiness is statistically abnormal, consists of a cluster of symptoms, is associated with a range of cognitive abnormalities and probably reflects the abnormal functioning of the central nervous system."

Yale University's June Gruber pointed out that "extreme happiness" can lead to a lack of negative emotions, which in turn leads to dangerous risk-taking and a "more severe illness course for mania." A lack of negative emotions is also typical of psychopaths, who don't feel remorse for antisocial behavior.

. . . Less Prepared to Fight or Flee

Gruber and her colleagues also pointed out that negative emotions lead to physiological changes that prepare the body to take action—for example, our heart rate increases when we feel fear, so that we can fight or flee. But if a person lacks these negative emotions, they "may be at a disadvantage," the researchers concluded, "because their bodies are not as well prepared to fight." Gruber added that a "cheerful person may be slower than a fearful person to detect a potential threat in the environment."

. . . Selfish

Through a trio of experiments, researchers at the University of New South Wales in Sydney, Australia, found that those in better moods tend to be less fair than those feeling sad. Using a "dictator game" that gave subjects the option to allocate scarce resources to themselves and to others as they saw fit, the researchers found that a good mood led to more selfish behavior. The reason? The researchers suggested that those who are feeling good are more focused on themselves, while those in a bad mood are more focused on the external—and are more sensitive to social norms.

. . . Worse at Negotiating

Whether asking for a raise or bargaining with a contractor, effective negotiations strike a balance between two or more people's differing interests—and usually leave everyone feeling a bit unhappy, but better than if they'd gotten nothing. But entering a negotiation in a good mood might actually hurt your chances of getting the best deal.

Researchers at the University of Amsterdam in the Netherlands tested this hypothesis in an experiment that charged participants to try to sell a consignment of mobile phones to an unseen buyer (actually a computer program) at the highest price possible. Before beginning the negotiation, the sellers were given statements about "the intentions of the buyer"—statements that reflected either their anger or happiness. The sellers who thought they were dealing with a happy opponent made the highest demands and gave the smallest concessions. Those who believed the seller to be angry made the lowest demands and asked for the largest concessions. The researchers expanded this out in a second experiment, which replicated the findings that participants with angry opponents placed lower demands on them.

. . . Poorer and Less Educated

Three researchers who have done much in the field of happiness research—Shigehiro Oishi, Ed Diener, and Richard E. Lucas—tackled the question of whether people can be too happy. They drew on vast amounts of data pulled from four large longitudinal surveys, a huge cross-sectional survey, and more, which added up to more than

100,000 respondents. They found that those who experience moderate levels of happiness (rather than the highest) are the top performers when it comes to income, education, and other areas.

Some of the reasons the researchers suggested: If you're completely happy with the current condition of things, you are unlikely to push yourself toward greater achievements in career and education. On a national or global level, individuals who are satisfied with the current state of the world are less likely to attempt to enact change or get involved in politics or activism.

But in the same study, when looking at relationships and volunteer work, the researchers found that the ultrahappy performed the best. It seems when it comes to making friends, there is no such thing as being *too* happy. They concluded that "the optimal mindset for an intimate relationship might be to see mostly the positive aspects of the partner and relationship, whereas the optimal mindset for income, education, and political participation might be to simultaneously consider the empty part of the glass as well as the fullness of it."

Getting Angry Has Its Perks

Sometimes, to win an argument, it can help to get a bit angry. And sometimes getting angry can be healthy for you. That was among the findings of a study of 175 people in which the participants role-played exercises. They would be either confrontational (playing a police officer interrogating a suspect) or collaborative. Before taking part in the role playing, the subjects chose which type of music they preferred to listen to for a given scenario—tunes aimed at making them feel angry, happy, or neutral.

Those who chose to listen to the angry music before getting confrontational—opting for a soundtrack that would help put them in the appropriate mood—were found to have greater levels of life satisfaction and networks of social support compared to those who preferred to feel happy or neutral before the argument. The researchers concluded that those who want to feel unpleasant emotions when they are useful might end up being happier overall.

· *Don't be afraid to break out a little fury during an argument.*

What Doesn't Kill You . . .

Experiencing a high level of adversity can have many long-term detrimental effects on a person, including lower life satisfaction and post-traumatic stress symptoms. But researchers have also found that some adversity can have lifelong emotional benefits. In a multi-year study, a team of researchers found that people with a history of *some* adversity actually reported better mental health and well-being than both those with *high* levels of adversity and those with none at all. The researchers attributed this to the greater levels of resilience built up by these individuals over time, allowing them to be less affected by more recent adverse events.

· *Write down some of the difficulties you've faced in your life and how you have been able to recover and grow from the adversity.*

Don't Fake It

For you to enjoy the many benefits of happiness—or for your happiness to make a positive impact on others—the happiness must be genuine. Researchers have found that feigned happiness (specifically, a fake smile) creates fewer positive impressions on those viewing it than authentic happiness. In an experiment from the University of California, San Francisco, a group of subjects was shown videos of people making real smiles and others making posed ones. There is a particular muscle movement surrounding the eye that can indicate that a smile is authentic (famously isolated by French anatomist G. B. Duchenne de Boulogne), and that is accepted as a measurement tool in determining whether a smile is real or fake.

Subjects who watched the videos could distinguish between the two types of smiles in as many as 81 percent of the cases. "A person is seen as more positive when they display an enjoyment smile compared with when they display a nonenjoyment smile," the researchers concluded, adding that those genuine smiles "were more accurately distinguished" from fake smiles and created greater positive impressions on observers.

Negative Is Smarter Than Positive

We have a tendency to see people who use negative language as smarter than those who use positive language. To investigate this, Harvard Business School professor Teresa Amabile wrote two identical reviews for a nonexistent book, making changes in ten places where either negative or positive words were inserted. Subjects believed that the negative reviewers had more literary expertise than the positive reviewers.

· *If you're generally a happy person, when writing or making an argument, slip in a bit of negativity to make an impression of more astuteness.*

Bad Is Stronger Than Good

For better or worse, negative life events make a stronger impact on us than positive events. Researchers have found that individuals with high levels of positive emotion tend to neglect important threats and dangers. In their article titled (naturally) "Bad Is

Stronger Than Good," researchers from Case Western Reserve University and Vrije Universiteit Amsterdam (Free University of Amsterdam) looked at why, with "hardly any exceptions," bad tends to trump good in our lives. They pointed out that bad parents, bad experiences, and bad meals all leave a greater impact on our lives than good ones. Losing money has been found to cause more distress than gaining money causes joy. We even make stronger facial expressions when reacting to an unpleasant odor than to a pleasant one.

The researchers suggested that being sensitive to bad things serves evolutionary purposes: making us avoid dangers, identify threats, and adapt and improve. While bad outcomes alert us that things need to change, good ones indicate that they do not. Our survival instinct leads us to worry about potentially negative outcomes rather than consider the potential greatness of positive outcomes. So, if you take one message away from this book, know that even bad things can help you be happier in the long run.

WHERE TO FIND THE SCIENCE

1: What Is Happiness?

Two Types of Happiness

Ed Diener and R. E. Lucas, "Personality and Subjective Well-Being," in D. Kahneman, Ed Diener, and N. Schwarz, Well-Being: Foundations of Hedonic Psychology *(New York: Russell Sage Foundation, 1999), 213–29.*

Ed Diener et al., "New Measures of Well-Being," in Assessing Well-Being, *ed. Ed Diener (New York: Springer, 2009), 247–66.*

Be Your True Self

Alan S. Waterman, "Two Conceptions of Happiness: Contrasts of Personal Expressiveness (Eudaimonia) and Hedonic Enjoyment," Journal of Personality and Social Psychology *64, no. 4 (1993): 678–691.*

Focus on the 40 Percent

Kristina M. DeNeve and Harris Cooper, "The Happy Personality: A Meta-Analysis of 137 Personality Traits and Subjective Well-Being," Psychological Bulletin *124, no. 2 (1998): 197–229.*

Sonja Lyubomirsky, The How of Happiness: A Scientific Approach to Getting the Life You Want *(New York: Penguin, 2008).*

2: Happy at Work

Ask: Why Are You Doing This?

Kennon M. Sheldon and Andrew J. Elliot, "Goal Striving, Need Satisfaction, and Longitudinal Well-Being: The Self-Concordance Model," Journal of Personality and Social Psychology *76, no. 3 (1999): 482–97.*

It's Not About the Paycheck

David Lykken and Auke Tellegen, "Happiness Is a Stochastic Phenomenon," Psychological Science *7, no. 3 (1996): 186–89.*

Daniel Kahneman and Angus Deaton, "High Income Improves Evaluation of Life but Not Emotional Well-Being," Proceedings of the National Academy of Sciences *107, no. 38 (2010): 16489–93.*

Andrew E. Clark and Andrew J. Oswald, "Satisfaction and Comparison Income," Journal of Public Economics *61, no. 3 (1996): 359–81.*

It's Not Even About a Really Big Paycheck

Ed Diener and Martin E. P. Seligman, "Beyond Money: Toward an Economy of Well-Being," Psychological Science in the Public Interest *5, no. 1 (2004): 1–31.*

Track Your Progress
C. Hoppmann and P. Klumb, "Daily Goal Pursuits Predict Cortisol Secretion and Mood States in Employed Parents with Preschool Children," Psychosomatic Medicine 68, no. 6: 887–94, https://doi.org/10.1097/01.psy.0000238232.46870.f1

Encourage Autonomy
Richard M. Ryan and Christina Frederick, "On Energy, Personality, and Health: Subjective Vitality as a Dynamic Reflection of Well-Being," Journal of Personality 65, no. 3 (1997): 529–65.

Show Your Happiness
Barry M. Staw, Robert I. Sutton, and Lisa H. Pelled, "Employee Positive Emotion and Favorable Outcomes at the Workplace," Organization Science 5, no. 1 (1994): 51–71.

Ditch Contracts
Deepak Malhotra and J. Keith Murnighan, "The Effects of Contracts on Interpersonal Trust," Administrative Science Quarterly 47, no. 3 (2002): 534–59.

Personalize Your Space
Craig Knight and S. Alexander Haslam, "The Relative Merits of Lean, Enriched, and Empowered Offices: An Experimental Examination of the Impact of Workspace Management Strategies on Well-Being and Productivity," Journal of Experimental Psychology: Applied 16, no. 2 (2010): 158–72.

Get Plants
Marlon Nieuwenhuis et al., "The Relative Benefits of Green Versus Lean Office Space: Three Field Experiments," Journal of Experimental Psychology: Applied 20, no. 3 (2014): 199–214.

Walk to Work, or Get a Bike
Evelyne St-Louis et al., "The Happy Commuter: A Comparison of Commuter Satisfaction Across Modes," Transportation Research Part F: Traffic Psychology and Behaviour 26, part A (2014): 160–70.

Write Down Meaningful Moments
Shawn Achor, "Positive Intelligence," Harvard Business Review 90, no. 1 (2012): 100–102.

Giada Di Stefano et al., "Making Experience Count: The Role of Reflection in Individual Learning," Harvard Business School NOM Unit Working Paper, no. 14-093 (2016).

Focus on Strengths
Susan Sorenson, "How Employees' Strengths Make Your Company Stronger," Gallup News, February 20, 2014.

Craft Your Job
Amy Wrzesniewski, Justin M. Berg, and Jane E. Dutton, "Managing Yourself: Turn the Job You Have into the Job You Want," Harvard Business Review 88, no. 6 (2010): 114–17.

Take a Proper Break
John P. Trougakos and Ivona Hideg, "Momentary Work Recovery: The Role of Within-Day Work Breaks," Current Perspectives on Job-Stress Recovery (Researh in Occupational Stress and Well-Being, 7) (Bingley, UK: Emerald Group Publishing Limited, 2009): 37–84.

. . . For 17 Minutes Off, 52 Minutes On
Derek Thompson, "A Formula for Perfect Productivity: Work for 52 Minutes, Break for 17," The Atlantic, September 17, 2014, https://www.theatlantic.com/business/archive/2014/09/science-tells-you-how-many-minutes-should-you-take-a-break-for-work-17/380369/

. . . Or for 5 Minutes Off, 25 Minutes On

Francesco Cirillo, "The Pomodoro Technique (The Pomodoro)," Agile Processes in Software Engineering and Extreme Programming 54, no. 2 (2006).

Don't Eat Lunch at Your Desk

John P. Trougakos et al., "Lunch Breaks Unpacked: The Role of Autonomy as a Moderator of Recovery During Lunch," Academy of Management Journal 57, no. 2 (2014): 405-21.

Don't Become a Lawyer

Martin E. P. Seligman, Paul R. Verkuil, and Terry H. Kang, "Why Lawyers Are Unhappy," Cardozo Law Review 23, no. 1 (2001): 33-54.

William W. Eaton et al., "Occupations and the Prevalence of Major Depressive Disorder," Journal of Occupational and Environmental Medicine 32, no. 11 (1990): 1079-87.

. . . Unless You Take a Pay Cut

Lawrence S. Krieger and Kennon M. Sheldon, "What Makes Lawyers Happy? Transcending the Anecdotes with Data from 6200 Lawyers," George Washington University Law Review 83, no. 2 (2015): 554-627.

What Are the Happiest Jobs

CareerBliss, "The Happiest Jobs in 2017," Forbes, https://www.forbes.com/ pictures/58c6d2f231358e1a35ace4cf/the-happiest-jobs-in-2017/#24851d8b6a89

Working Less Won't Make You Happier

Danish Ministry of the Environment, Happiness Research Institute, "Job Satisfaction Index 2017," https://docs.wixstatic.com/ugd/928487_f752364b0a43488c8c767532c0de4926.pdf

Ruut Veenhoven, "Informed Pursuit of Happiness: What We Should Know, Do Know and Can Get to Know," Journal of Happiness Studies 16, no. 4 (2015): 1035-71.

Don't Retire Early

Ruut Veenhoven, Findings on Happiness & Retirement (World Database of Happiness, Subject code R3, 2009), http://www.academia.edu/27197961/Findings_on_Happiness_ and_Retirement

Susan Rohwedder and Robert J. Willis, "Mental Retirement," The Journal of Economic Perspectives: A Journal of the American Economic Association 24, no. 1 (2010): 119-38.

Gina Kolata, "Taking Early Retirement May Retire Memory, Too," New York Times, October 11, 2010.

Meditate

Lorenza S. Colzato, Ayca Ozturk, and Bernhard Hommel, "Meditate to Create: The Impact of Focused-Attention and Open-Monitoring Training on Convergent and Divergent Thinking," Frontiers in Psychology 3 (2012): 116.

Take Up Yoga

N. Hartfiel et al., "Yoga for Reducing Perceived Stress and Back Pain at Work," Occupational Medicine 62, no. 8 (2012): 606-12.

3: Happy at Play

Sandie McHugh et al., "Everyday Leisure and Happiness in Worktown: A Comparison of 1938 and 2014," World Leisure Journal 58, no. 4 (2016): 276-84.

Choose Happiness-Boosting Activities
Miao Wang and M. C. Sunny Wong, "Happiness and Leisure Across Countries: Evidence from International Survey Data," Journal of Happiness Studies *15, no. 1 (2014): 85–118.*

Make Contacts
Wang and Wong, "Happiness and Leisure Across Countries."

Get Outside
Carey Knecht, "Urban Nature and Well-Being: Some Empirical Support and Design Implications," Berkeley Planning Journal *17, no. 1 (2004).*

Head to the Park
Liisa Tyrväinen et al., "The Influence of Urban Green Environments on Stress Relief Measures: A Field Experiment," Journal of Environmental Psychology *38 (2014): 1–9.*
Knecht, "Urban Nature and Well-Being."

. . . Or Sit by a Window
Roger S. Ulrich et al., "Stress Recovery During Exposure to Natural and Urban Environments," Journal of Environmental Psychology *11, no. 3 (1991): 201–30.*

Join a Sport
Haifang Huang and Brad R. Humphreys, "Sports Participation and Happiness: Evidence from US Microdata," Journal of Economic Psychology *33, no. 4 (2012): 776–93.*
Shea M. Balish, Dan Conacher, and Lori Dithurbide, "Sport and Recreation Are Associated with Happiness Across Countries," Research Quarterly for Exercise and Sport *87, no. 4 (2016): 382–88.*

Make Leisure a Habit
Andrew W. Bailey and Irene K. Fernando, "Routine and Project-Based Leisure, Happiness, and Meaning in Life," Journal of Leisure Research *(2012): 139–54.*

Value Time over Money
Hal E. Hershfield, Cassie Mogilner, and Uri Barnea, "People Who Choose Time Over Money Are Happier," Social Psychological and Personality Science *7, no. 7 (2016): 697–706.*

Buy Experiences, Not Things
Ryan T. Howell, Paulina Pchelin, and Ravi Iyer, "The Preference for Experiences Over Possessions: Measurement and Construct Validation of the Experiential Buying Tendency Scale," Journal of Positive Psychology *7, no. 1 (2012): 57–71.*
Leaf Van Boven and Thomas Gilovich, "To Do or to Have? That Is the Question," Journal of Personality and Social Psychology *85, no. 6 (2003): 1193–202.*

Take Eight-Day Vacations
Jessica De Bloom, Sabine A. E. Geurts, and Michiel A. J. Kompier, "Vacation (After-) Effects on Employee Health and Well-Being, and the Role of Vacation Activities, Experiences and Sleep," Journal of Happiness Studies *14, no. 2 (2013): 613–33.*

Plan Vacations Earlier
Jeroen Nawijn et al., "Vacationers Happier, but Most Not Happier After a Holiday," Applied Research in Quality of Life *5, no. 1 (2010): 35–47.*

Have Fun First
Ed O'Brien and Ellen Roney, "Worth the Wait? Leisure Can Be Just as Enjoyable with Work Left Undone," Psychological Science *28, no. 7 (2017): 1000–1015, https://doi.org/10.1177/0956797617701749.*

You're More Competent on the Weekend

Richard M. Ryan, Jessey H. Bernstein, and Kirk Warren Brown, "Weekends, Work, and Well-Being: Psychological Need Satisfactions and Day of the Week Effects on Mood, Vitality, and Physical Symptoms," Journal of Social and Clinical Psychology 29, no. 1 (2010): 95–122.

Go with the Flow

Jeanne Nakamura and Mihály Csíkszentmihályi, "Flow Theory and Research," in Handbook of Positive Psychology, ed. C. R. Snyder and Shane J. Lopez (New York: Oxford University Press, 2009): 195–206.

Flow in Teams

Charles J. Walker, "Experiencing Flow: Is Doing It Together Better Than Doing It Alone?," Journal of Positive Psychology 5, no. 1 (2010): 3–11.

Find an Adventure

Christopher D. Jones et al., "Validation of the Flow Theory in an On-Site Whitewater Kayaking Setting," Journal of Leisure Research 32, no. 2 (2000): 247–61.

Knit . . . or Quilt

Jill Riley, Betsan Corkhill, and Clare Morris, "The Benefits of Knitting for Personal and Social Wellbeing in Adulthood: Findings from an International Survey," British Journal of Occupational Therapy 76, no. 2 (2013): 50–57.

Emily L. Burt and Jacqueline Atkinson, "The Relationship Between Quilting and Wellbeing," Journal of Public Health 34, no. 1 (2011): 54–59.

Get Playful

René T. Proyer, "The Well-Being of Playful Adults: Adult Playfulness, Subjective Well-Being, Physical Well-Being, and the Pursuit of Enjoyable Activities," European Journal of Humour Research 1, no. 1 (2013): 84–98.

Crack a Joke

Paul McGhee, Humor as Survival Training For a Stressed-Out World: The 7 Humor Habits Program *(Bloomington, IN: Author House, 2010).*

Shelley A. Crawford and Nerina J. Caltabiano, "Promoting Emotional Well-Being Through the Use of Humour," Journal of Positive Psychology 6, no. 3 (2011): 237–52.

. . . But Not at Someone Else's Expense

Thomas E. Ford, Katelyn A. McCreight, and Kyle Richardson, "Affective Style, Humor Styles and Happiness," Europe's Journal of Psychology 10, no. 3 (2014): 451–63.

Limit Your Options

Sheena S. Iyengar and Mark R. Lepper, "When Choice Is Demotivating: Can One Desire Too Much of a Good Thing?," Journal of Personality and Social Psychology 79, no. 6 (2000): 995–1006.

Become a Bar Regular

Robin Dunbar, "Friends on Tap: The Role of Pubs at the Heart of the Community," Oxford: Campaign for Real Ale, http://www.camra.org.uk/documents/10180/36197/ Friends+on+Tap/2c68585b-e47d-42ca-bda6-5d6b3e4c0110

Listen with Intention

Yuna L. Ferguson and Kennon M. Sheldon, "Trying to Be Happier Really Can Work: Two Experimental Studies," Journal of Positive Psychology 8, no. 1 (2013): 23–33.

Cool Down

Yoshiro Tsutsui, "Weather and Individual Happiness," Weather, Climate, and Society *5, no. 1 (2013): 70–82.*

Do Something for Someone Else

Dylan Wiwad and Lara B. Aknin, "Self-Focused Motives Undermine the Emotional Rewards of Recalled Prosocial Behavior" (2017), https://doi.org/10.17605/OSF.IO/96QWA

4: Happy in Love

Five Is the Magic Number

J. M. Gottman, What Predicts Divorce? The Relationship Between Marital Processes and Marital Outcomes *(Hillsdale, NJ: Lawrence Erlbaum Associates, 1994).*

Wait at Least a Month for Sex

Sharon Sassler, Fenaba R. Addo, and Daniel T. Lichter, "The Tempo of Sexual Activity and Later Relationship Quality," Journal of Marriage and Family *74, no. 4 (2012): 708–25.*

Do a Daily Debrief

Terri L. Orbuch, 5 Simple Steps to Take Your Marriage from Good to Great *(New York: Delacorte Press, 2009), 88–89.*

Repair Your Relationship House

John Gottman and Julie Gottman, "The Natural Principles of Love," Journal of Family Theory & Review *9, no. 1 (2017): 7–26.*

Seek Out "Bids"

Kristin Ohlson, "The Einstein of Love," Psychology Today, *September 1, 2015.*

Celebrate Good News

Shelly L. Gable, Gian C. Gonzaga, and Amy Strachman, "Will You Be There for Me When Things Go Right? Supportive Responses to Positive Event Disclosures," Journal of Personality and Social Psychology *91, no. 5 (2006): 904–17.*

Jill M. Logan and Rebecca J. Cobb, "Benefits of Capitalization in Newlyweds: Predicting Marital Satisfaction and Depression Symptoms," Journal of Social and Clinical Psychology *35, no. 2 (2016): 87–106.*

Celebrate Tough Times, Too

J. Flora and C. Segrin, "Relationship Development in Dating Couples: Implications for Relational Satisfaction and Loneliness," Journal of Social and Personal Relationships *17, no. 6 (2000): 811–25.*

Get More Sleep

American Academy of Sleep Medicine, "Poor Sleep Is Associated with Lower Relationship Satisfaction in Both Women and Men," ScienceDaily, *June 15, 2009.*

Friends' Relationships Are Important, Too

Rose McDermott, James H. Fowler, and Nicholas A. Christakis, "Breaking Up Is Hard to Do, Unless Everyone Else Is Doing It Too: Social Network Effects on Divorce in a Longitudinal Sample," Social Forces *92, no. 2 (2013): 491–519.*

Raise Your Credit Score

Jane Dokko, Geng Li, and Jessica Hayes, "Credit Scores and Committed Relationships," FEDS Working Paper No. 2015-081, *http://dx.doi.org/10.17016/FEDS.2015.081*

Create a Division of Labor

Wendy Klein, Carolina Izquierdo, and Thomas N. Bradbury, "Working Relationships: Communicative Patterns and Strategies Among Couples in Everyday Life," Qualitative Research in Psychology *4, no. 1-2 (2007): 29-47.*

Rethink What You're Getting from Sex

A. Gewirtz-Meydan and R. Finzi-Dottan, "Sexual Satisfaction Among Couples: The Role of Attachment Orientation and Sexual Motives," Journal of Sex Research *(February 2017): 1-13, https://doi.org/10.1080/00224499.2016.1276880.*

Seek Similar Spending Habits

Scott I. Rick, Deborah A. Small, and Eli J. Finkel, "Fatal (Fiscal) Attraction: Spendthrifts and Tightwads in Marriage," Journal of Marketing Research *48, no. 2 (2011): 228-37.*

Say "We"

Benjamin H. Seider et al., "We Can Work It Out: Age Differences in Relational Pronouns, Physiology, and Behavior in Marital Conflict," Psychology *and Aging 24, no. 3 (2009): 604-13.*

Turn On a Sappy Romance

S. A. Vannier and L. F. O'Sullivan, "Passion, Connection and Destiny: How Romantic Expectations Help Predict Satisfaction and Commitment in Young Adults' Dating Relationships," Journal of Social and Personal Relationships *34 (2017): 235-57, https://doi .org/10.1177/0265407516631156*

Put On Those Rose-Colored Glasses

Sandra L. Murray et al., "Tempting Fate or Inviting Happiness? Unrealistic Idealization Prevents the Decline of Marital Satisfaction," Psychological Science. *22, no. 5 (2011): 619-26, https://doi.org/10.1177/0956797611403155*

Punch Up Your "How We Met" Story

Kim Therese Buehlman, John Mordechai Gottman, and Lynn Fainsilber Katz, "How a Couple Views Their Past Predicts Their Future: Predicting Divorce from an Oral History Interview," Journal of Family Psychology *5, no. 3-4 (1992): 295-318.*

Maintain Friendships Outside the Marriage

Geoffrey L. Greif and Kathleen Holtz Deal, Two Plus Two: Couples and Their Couple Friendships *(New York: Routledge, 2012).*

Change Up Date Night

Arthur Aron, Christina C. Norman, and Elaine N. Aron, "Shared Self-Expanding Activities as a Means of Maintaining and Enhancing Close Romantic Relationships," in Close Romantic Relationships: Maintenance and Enhancement, *ed. John H. Harvey and Amy Wenzel (Mahwah, NJ: Lawrence Erlbaum Associates, 2001): 47-66.*

Keep a Journal Handy

Ting Zhang et al., "A 'Present' for the Future: The Unexpected Value of Rediscovery," Psychological Science *25, no. 10 (2014): 1851-60.*

Make Time for Sex

Tara Parker-Pope, "Sex and the Long-Term Relationship," New York Times, *March 22, 2011.*

5: Happy at Home

Brighten Up

Ping Dong, Xun Huang, and Chen-Bo Zhong, "Ray of Hope: Hopelessness Increases Preferences for Brighter Lighting," Social Psychological and Personality Science 6, no. 1 (2015): 84–91.

Rikard Küller et al., "The Impact of Light and Colour on Psychological Mood: A Cross-Cultural Study of Indoor Work Environments," Ergonomics 49, no. 14 (2006): 1496–1507.

Beware Blue Light

M. Boubekri et al., "Impact of Workplace Daylight Exposure on Sleep, Physical Activity, and Quality of Life," SLEEP (American Academy of Sleep Medicine) 36 (2013): 30.

"Blue Light Has a Dark Side," Harvard Health Letter, September 2, 2015.

Create a Fake Sun

Virginie Gabel et al., "Effects of Artificial Dawn and Morning Blue Light on Daytime Cognitive Performance, Well-Being, Cortisol and Melatonin Levels," Chronobiology International 30, no. 8 (2013): 988–97.

Place Your Desk Sideways to the Window

Mohamed Boubekri, Robert B. Hull, and Lester L. Boyer, "Impact of Window Size and Sunlight Penetration on Office Workers' Mood and Satisfaction: A Novel Way of Assessing Sunlight," Environment and Behavior 23, no. 4 (1991): 474–93.

Be Messy—in Creative Places

Kathleen Vohs, Aparna Labroo, and Ravi Dhar, "The Upside of Messy Surroundings: Cueing Divergent Thinking, Problem Solving, and Increasing Creativity," NA -Advances in Consumer Research (Association for Consumer Research) 44 (2016): 264–68.

But Skip the Abstract Art

Roger S. Ulrich, "Effects of Interior Design on Wellness: Theory and Recent Scientific Research," Journal of Health Care Interior Design 3 (1991): 97–109.

Warm Up Your Walls

Kemal Yildirim, Kemal, M. Lutfi Hidayetoglu, and Aysen Capanoglu, "Effects of Interior Colors on Mood and Preference: Comparisons of Two Living Rooms," Perceptual and Motor Skills 112, no. 2 (2011): 509–24.

Raise the Roof

Joan Meyers-Levy and Rui Zhu, "The Influence of Ceiling Height: The Effect of Priming on the Type of Processing That People Use," Journal of Consumer Research 34, no. 2 (2007): 174–86.

Love Those Curves

Moshe Bar and Maital Neta, "Humans Prefer Curved Visual Objects," Psychological Science 17, no. 8 (2006): 645–48.

Place a Notepad and Trash Can Near the Mirror

Pablo Briñol et al., "Treating Thoughts as Material Objects Can Increase or Decrease Their Impact on Evaluation," Psychological Science 24, no. 1 (2013): 41–47.

If You Build It . . .

Michael I. Norton, Daniel Mochon, and Dan Ariely, "The IKEA Effect: When Labor Leads to Love," Journal of Consumer Psychology 22, no. 3 (2012): 453–60.

Get Some Flowers

Jeannette Haviland-Jones et al., "An Environmental Approach to Positive Emotion: Flowers," Evolutionary Psychology *3, no. 1 (2005): 104–32, https://doi .org/10.1177/147470490500300109*

Enjoy the View

Ernest O. Moore, "A Prison Environment's Effect on Health Care Service Demands," Journal of Environmental Systems *11, no. 1 (1981): 17–34.*

Roger Ulrich, "View Through a Window May Influence Recovery," Science *224, no. 4647 (1984): 420–21.*

Carolyn M. Tennessen and Bernadine Cimprich, "Views to Nature: Effects on Attention," Journal of Environmental Psychology *15, no. 1 (1995): 77–85.*

When You Feel Bad, Reach Out and Touch Something

Dan King and Chris Janiszewski, "Affect-Gating," Journal of Consumer Research, *38, no. 4 (2011): 697–711.*

Create a "Relaxation Room"

Karen J. Sherman et al., "Effectiveness of Therapeutic Massage for Generalized Anxiety Disorder: A Randomized Controlled Trial," Depression and Anxiety *27, no. 5 (2010): 441–50.*

Turn Off the TV

John P. Robinson and Steven Martin, "What Do Happy People Do?," Social Indicators Research *89, no. 3 (2008): 565–71.*

Get a Savings Jar

Aaron C. Weidman and Elizabeth W. Dunn, "The Unsung Benefits of Material Things: Material Purchases Provide More Frequent Momentary Happiness Than Experiential Purchases," Social Psychological and Personality Science *7, no. 4 (2016): 390–99.*

Reconsider That Open-Concept Kitchen

Kimberly A. Rollings and Nancy M. Wells, "Effects of Floor Plan Openness on Eating Behaviors," Environment and Behavior *49, no. 6 (2016): 663–84, https://doi .org/10.1177/0013916516661822.*

Move Closer to Work

Lars E. Olsson et al., "Happiness and Satisfaction with Work Commute," Social Indicators Research *111, no. 1 (2013): 255–63.*

Rent Instead of Buy

Rosie Murray-West, "What Makes a Happy Home?," The Telegraph, *March 27, 2017, http:// www.telegraph.co.uk/tv/rich-house-poor-house/what-makes-a-happy-home/*

Reduce, Reuse, and Smile

Jeffrey C. Jacob and Merlin B. Brinkerhoff, "Mindfulness and Subjective Well-Being in the Sustainability Movement: A Further Elaboration of Multiple Discrepancies Theory," Social Indicators Research *46, no. 3 (1999): 341–68.*

Jing Jian Xiao and Haifeng Li, "Sustainable Consumption and Life Satisfaction," Social Indicators Research *104, no. 2 (2011): 323–29.*

Xavier Landes et al., Sustainable Happiness: Why Waste Prevention May Lead to an Increase in Quality of Life *(Danish Ministry of the Environment, Happiness Research Institute, 2015).*

6: Happy in Friendship

150 Is the Magic Number
R. Dunbar, How Many Friends Does One Person Need?: Dunbar's Number and Other Evolutionary Quirks *(Cambridge, MA: Harvard University Press, 2010).*

Layer Up
Dunbar, R. I. M. "Mind the Gap: Or Why Humans Aren't Just Great Apes," Proceedings of the British Academy *154 (2008): 403-423.*

Seek Out Happy Friends–and Acquaintances
James H. Fowler and Nicholas A. Christakis, "Dynamic Spread of Happiness in a Large Social Network," BMJ *337 (2008): a2338.*

Smell a Happy Person
Jasper H. B. de Groot et al., "A Sniff of Happiness," Psychological Science *26, no. 6 (2015): 684-700.*

Spend More Time Together
Harry T. Reis et al., "Familiarity Does Indeed Promote Attraction in Live Interaction," Journal of Personality and Social Psychology *101, no. 3 (2011): 557.*

Get Personal
Arthur Aron et al., "The Experimental Generation of Interpersonal Closeness: A Procedure and Some Preliminary Findings," Personality and Social Psychology Bulletin *23, no. 4 (1997): 363-77.*

Cultivate Engaged Conversations
Harry Weger Jr. et al., "The Relative Effectiveness of Active Listening in Initial Interactions," International Journal of Listening, *28, no.1 (2014), 13-31.*

Less Can Be More . . .
M. Demir and L. A. Weitekamp, "I Am So Happy 'Cause Today I Found My Friend: Friendship and Personality as Predictors of Happiness," Journal of Happiness Studies, *8, no. 2 (2007): 181-211.*

. . . But Acquaintances Are Key
G. M. Sandstrom and E. W. Dunn, "Social Interactions and Well-Being: The Surprising Power of Weak Ties," Personality & Social Psychology Bulletin *40, no. 7 (2014): 910-22.*
Demir and Weitekamp, "I Am So Happy."
J. E. Perry-Smith, "Social Yet Creative: The Role of Social Relationships in Facilitating Individual Creativity," Academy of Management Journal *49, no. 1 (2006): 85-101.*

Give . . .
Lara B. Akins, J. Kiley Hamlin, and Elizabeth W. Dunn, "Giving Leads to Happiness in Young Children" (June 14, 2012), http://journals.plos.org/plosone/article?id=10.1371/journal .pone.0039211

Turn a Workplace Acquaintance into a Great Friend
Patricia M. Sias and Daniel J. Cahill, "The Development of Peer Friendships in the Workplace," Western Journal of Communication *62, no. 3 (1998): 273-99.*

. . . Experiences . . .
Cindy Chan and Cassie Mogilner, "Experiential Gifts Foster Stronger Social Relationships Than Material Gifts," Journal of Consumer Research *43, no. 6 (2017): 913-31.*

. . . But Don't Be Too Generous

Craig D. Parks and Asako B. Stone, "The Desire to Expel Unselfish Members from the Group," Journal of Personality and Social Psychology *99, no. 2 (2010): 303.*

Climb the "Local Ladder"

C. Anderson et al., "The Local-Ladder Effect: Social Status and Subjective Well-Being," Psychological Science, *23 (2012): 764-71, https://doi.org/10.1177/0956797611434537*

Complain with Purpose

R. Kowalski et al., "Pet Peeves and Happiness: How Do Happy People Complain?," Journal of Social Psychology *154, no. 4 (2014): 278-82.*

Follow the Five Steps of Emotional Intelligence

Daniel Goleman, "How to Be Emotionally Intelligent," New York Times, *April 12, 2015.*

Sample a Complaint Sandwich

E. Demerouti and R. Cropanzano, "The Buffering Role of Sportsmanship on the Effects of Daily Negative Events," European Journal of Work and Organizational Psychology, *26, no. 2 (2017): 263-74.*

Guy Winch, The Squeaky Wheel *(New York: Walker & Company, 2011).*

Apologize Effectively

R. Fehr and M. Gelfand, "When Apologies Work: How Matching Apology Components to Victims' Self-Construals Facilitates Forgiveness," Organizational Behavior and Human Decision Processes *113, no. 1 (2010): 37-50.*

Make Friends Feel Competent

Meliksah Demir and Ingrid Davidson, "Toward a Better Understanding of the Relationship Between Friendship and Happiness: Perceived Responses to Capitalization Attempts, Feelings of Mattering, and Satisfaction of Basic Psychological Needs in Same-Sex Best Friendships as Predictors of Happiness," Journal of Happiness Studies *14, no. 2 (2013): 525-50.*

Follow the Rules of Friendship

M. Argyle and M. Henderson, "The Rules of Friendship," Journal of Social and Personal Relationships *1, no. 2 (1984): 211-37.*

Don't Let a New Job Kill Old Friendships

D. L. Sollie and J. L. Fischer, "Career Entry Influences on Social Networks of Young Adults: A Longitudinal Study," Journal of Social Behavior & Personality *3, no. 4 (1988): 205-25.*

Watch Those Drinks

J. Thrul and E. Kuntsche, "The Impact of Friends on Young Adults' Drinking Over the Course of the Evening—An Event-Level Analysis," Addiction *110, no. 4 (2015): 619-26.*

7: Happy in Health

Ten Minutes Is Enough

Cheryl J. Hansen, Larry C. Stevens, and J. Richard Coast, "Exercise Duration and Mood State: How Much Is Enough to Feel Better?," Health Psychology *20, no. 4 (2001): 267-75.*

Skip the Gym

Thomas Bossmann et al., "The Association Between Short Periods of Everyday Life Activities and Affective States: A Replication Study Using Ambulatory Assessment," Frontiers in Psychology *4 (2013), https://doi.org/10.3389/fpsyg.2013.00102*

Feel Less Exhausted . . . by Working Out Longer

Courtney A. Rocheleau et al., "Moderators of the Relationship Between Exercise and Mood Changes: Gender, Exertion Level, and Workout Duration," Psychology & Health 19, no. 4 (2004): 491–506.

Seven (Minutes) to Succeed

Brett Klika and Chris Jordan, "High-Intensity Circuit Training Using Body Weight: Maximum Results with Minimal Investment," ACSM's Health & Fitness Journal 17, no. 3 (2013): 8–13.

Dehydration Can Be a Downer

Lawrence E. Armstrong et al., "Mild Dehydration Affects Mood in Healthy Young Women," Journal of Nutrition 142, no. 2 (2012): 382–88.

Watch Out for Dry Eyes

Motoko Kawashima et al., "Associations Between Subjective Happiness and Dry Eye Disease: A New Perspective from the Osaka Study," PLoS ONE 10, no. 4 (2015): e0123299.

Get Older

Nancy L. Galambos et al., "Up, Not Down: The Age Curve in Happiness from Early Adulthood to Midlife in Two Longitudinal Studies," Developmental Psychology 51, no. 11 (2015): 1664.

Filter Out the Negative

Laura L. Carstensen and Joseph A. Mikels, "At the Intersection of Emotion and Cognition: Aging and the Positivity Effect," Current Directions in Psychological Science 14, no. 3 (2005): 117–21.

Drink More Coffee

Erikka Loftfield and Neal D. Freedman, "Higher Coffee Consumption Is Associated with Lower Risk of All-Cause and Cause-Specific Mortality in Three Large Prospective Cohorts," Evidence-Based Medicine 21 no. 3 (2016): 108.

. . . Or Take a Break from Caffeine—Then Restart It

Merideth A. Addicott and Paul J. Laurienti, "A Comparison of the Effects of Caffeine Following Abstinence and Normal Caffeine Use," Psychopharmacology 207, no. 3 (2009): 423–31.

Eat Your Fruits and Vegetables

Redzo Mujcic and Andrew J. Oswald, "Evolution of Well-Being and Happiness After Increases in Consumption of Fruit and Vegetables," American Journal of Public Health 106, no. 8 (2016): 1504–10.

Grab Some Nuts

Almudena Sánchez-Villegas et al., "Mediterranean Dietary Pattern and Depression: The PREDIMED Randomized Trial," BMC Medicine 11, no. 208 (2013).

Get Your Zs

Andrea N. Goldstein and Matthew P. Walker, "The Role of Sleep in Emotional Brain Function," Annual Review of Clinical Psychology 10 (2014): 679–708.

Seven (Hours) to a Long Life

Daniel F. Kripke et al., "Mortality Associated with Sleep Duration and Insomnia," Archives of General Psychiatry 59 (2002): 131–36.

Skip the Sleeping Pills

Daniel F. Kripke et al., "Mortality Hazard Associated with Prescription Hypnotics," Biological Psychiatry 43, no. 9 (1998): 687–93.

If You Miss Sleep, You Can Get It Back

Hee-Jin Im et al., "Association Between Weekend Catch-Up Sleep and Lower Body Mass: Population-Based Study," Journal of Sleep and Sleep Disorders Research 40, no. 7 (2017): https://doi.org/ 10.1093/sleep/zsx089

Work Out with Friends

Arran Davis, Jacob Taylor, and Emma Cohen, "Social Bonds and Exercise: Evidence for a Reciprocal Relationship," PLoS ONE 10, no. 8 (2015): e0136705.

Eat Chocolate . . . but Be Mindful About It

Brian P. Meier, Sabrina W. Noll, and Oluwatobi J. Molokwu, "The Sweet Life: The Effect of Mindful Chocolate Consumption on Mood," Appetite 108 (2017): 21-27.

Competition Is More Motivating Than Encouragement

Jingwen Zhang et al., "Support or Competition? How Online Social Networks Increase Physical Activity: A Randomized Controlled Trial," Preventive Medicine Reports 4 (2016): 453-58.

Track Your Food

Lora E. Burke, Jing Wang, and Mary Ann Sevick, "Self-Monitoring in Weight Loss: A Systematic Review of the Literature," Journal of the American Dietetic Association 111, no. 1 (2011): 92-102.

. . . And Track Your Actions

Ta-Chien Chan et al., "ClickDiary: Online Tracking of Health Behaviors and Mood," Journal of Medical Internet Research 17, no. 6 (2015): e147, https://doi.org/10.2196/jmir.4315

Move—Right Now

Neal Lathia et al., "Happier People Live More Active Lives: Using Smartphones to Link Happiness and Physical Activity," PLoS ONE 12, no. 1 (2017): e0160589.

The Cure for the Common Cold Might be a Good Mood

Sheldon Cohen et al., "Positive Emotional Style Predicts Resistance to Illness After Experimental Exposure to Rhinovirus or Influenza A Virus," Psychosomatic Medicine 68, no. 6 (2006): 809-15.

Appreciate Your Body

Viren Swami et al., "Associations Between Women's Body Image and Happiness: Results of the YouBeauty.com Body Image Survey (YBIS)," Journal of Happiness Studies 16, no. 3 (2015): 705-18.

8: High-Tech Happiness

Ask: For What Are You Using the Internet?

C. F. Gordon, L. P. Juang, and M. Syed, "Internet Use and Well-Being Among College Students: Beyond Frequency of Use," Journal of College Student Development 48, no. 6 (2007): 674-88.

Beware Internet Addiction

R. W. Kubey, M. J. Lavin, and J. R. Barrows, "Internet Use and Collegiate Academic Performance Decrements: Early Findings," Journal of Communication 51, no. 2 (2001): 366-82.

Stop Apologizing

Thomas Jackson, Ray Dawson, and Darren Wilson, "Case Study: Evaluating the Effect of Email Interruptions Within the Workplace," Proceedings of Conference on Empirical Assessment in Software Engineering, Keele University, UK (2002): 3-7, https://dspace .lboro.ac.uk/2134/489

Dunbar's Number Works on Twitter

B. Gonçalves, N. Perra, and A. Vespignani, "Modeling Users' Activity on Twitter Networks: Validation of Dunbar's Number," PLoS ONE 6, no. 8 (2011): e22656.

Turn Off Your Social Networks

C. Coccia and C. A. Darling, "Having the Time of Their Life: College Student Stress, Dating and Satisfaction with Life," Stress and Health 32, no. 1 (2016): 28–35.

Don't Trust Apps to Find You Love

Samantha Joel, Paul W. Eastwick, and Eli J. Finkel, "Is Romantic Desire Predictable? Machine Learning Applied to Initial Romantic Attraction," Psychological Science 29 no. 10 (2017): 1478–89, https://doi.org/10.1177/0956797617714580

Take a Social Sabbatical

Morten Tromholt, "The Facebook Experiment: Quitting Facebook Leads to Higher Levels of Well-Being," Cyberpsychology, Behavior, and Social Networking 19, no. 11 (2016): 661–66.

Text for "Relationship Maintenance"

Lori Cluff Schade et al., "Using Technology to Connect in Romantic Relationships: Effects on Attachment, Relationship Satisfaction, and Stability in Emerging Adults," Journal of Couple and Relationship Therapy 12, no. 4 (2013): 314–38.

Talk, Don't Text, Over Long Distances

Lijuan Yin, "Communication Channels, Social Support and Satisfaction in Long Distance Romantic Relationships" (master's thesis, Georgia State University, 2009), https://scholarworks.gsu.edu/communication_theses/56

Texting Kills Your GPA

A. Lepp, J. E. Barkley, and A. C. Karpinski, "The Relationship Between Cell Phone Use, Academic Performance, Anxiety, and Satisfaction with Life in College Students," Computers in Human Behavior 31 (2014): 343–50.

Cell Phones Increase Anxiety

Lepp, Barkley, and Karpinski, "Relationship Between Cell Phone Use."

Keep It Personal

Moira Burke and Robert E. Kraut, "The Relationship Between Facebook Use and Well-Being Depends on Communication Type and Tie Strength," Journal of Computer-Mediated Communication 21, no. 4 (2016): 265–81.

Use Facebook to Build Offline Social Capital

N. B. Ellison, C. Steinfield, and C. Lampe, "The Benefits of Facebook 'Friends': Social Capital and College Students' Use of Online Social Network Sites," Journal of Computer-Mediated Communication 12, no. 4 (2007): 1143–68.

Stop Comparing, Start Appreciating

Erin A. Vogel et al., "Social Comparison, Social Media, and Self-Esteem," Psychology of Popular Media Culture 3, no. 4 (2014): 206–22.

Leon Festinger, "A Theory of Social Comparison Processes," Human Relations 7, no. 2 (1954): 117–40.

James Hamblin, "The Psychology of Healthy Facebook Use: No Comparing to Other Lives," The Atlantic, April 8, 2015.

Play More Video Games

Younbo Jung et al., "Games for a Better Life: Effects of Playing Wii Games on the Well-Being of Seniors in a Long-Term Care Facility," Proceedings of the Sixth Australasian Conference on Interactive Entertainment, 2009, https://doi.org/10.1145/1746050.1746055

Snap a Selfie

Yu Chen, Gloria Mark, and Sanna Ali, "Promoting Positive Affect Through Smartphone Photography," Psychology of Well-Being *6, no. 1 (2016): 8.*

More Radio and Less TV

B. S. Frey and C. Benesch, "TV, Time and Happiness," Homo Oeconomicus *25, no. 3/4(2008): 12.*

. . . Though Watching TV with a Significant Other Can Be Healthy

Sarah Gomillion et al., "Let's Stay Home and Watch TV: The Benefits of Shared Media Use for Close Relationships," Journal of Social and Personal Relationships *(2016): 1–20, https:// doi.org/10.1177/0265407516660388*

9: Finding Your Happy Place

Get Out of Town

Brian J. L. Berry and Adam Okulicz-Kozaryn, "An Urban-Rural Happiness Gradient," Urban Geography *32, no. 6 (2011): 871–83.*

. . . Or Do Cities Get a Bad Rap?

Edward Glaeser, Triumph of the City: How Our Greatest Invention Makes Us Richer, Smarter, Greener, Healthier, and Happier *(New York: Penguin Press, 2011).*

Measuring Quality of Life

Dimitris Ballas, "What Makes a 'Happy City'?," Cities *32 (2013): S39–S50.*

John L. Girt, "The Geography of Social Well-Being in the United States: An Introduction to Territorial Social Indicators," Social Indicators Research *1, no. 2 (1974): 257–59.*

Jennifer Roback, "Wages, Rents, and Amenities: Differences Among Workers and Regions," Economic Inquiry *26, no. 1 (1988): 23–41.*

Seek Social Support and Economic Stability

John F. Helliwell, Haifang Huang, and Shun Wang, "The Social Foundations of World Happiness," in World Happiness Report 2017 *(New York: Sustainable Development Solutions Network, 2017): 8–46.*

Give Europe a Look

Mercer's quality of living index, https://www.mercer.com/newsroom/2017-quality-of-living-survey.html

Equality Benefits All

Shigehiro Oishi, Selin Kesebir, and Ed Diener, "Income Inequality and Happiness," Psychological Science *22, no. 9 (2011): 1095–100.*

Richard Wilkinson and Kate Pickett, The Spirit Level: Why Equality Is Better For Everyone *(London: Penguin UK, 2010).*

Inequality Index

Wim Kalmijn and Ruut Veenhoven, "Index of Inequality-Adjusted Happiness (IAH) Improved: A Research Note," Journal of Happiness Studies *15, no. 6 (2014): 1259–65.*

Emotion Matters

Eunkook Suh et al., "The Shifting Basis of Life Satisfaction Judgments Across Cultures: Emotions Versus Norms," Journal of Personality and Social Psychology *74, no. 2 (1998): 482–93.*

Consider the Ideal Affect

Jeanne L. Tsai, "Ideal Affect: Cultural Causes and Behavioral Consequences," Perspectives on Psychological Science *2, no. 3 (2007): 242–59.*

Freedom Beats Money
Amartya Sen, Development as Freedom *(New York: Oxford University Press, 1999).*
Host a Sports Event
Georgios Kavetsos and Stefan Szymanski, "National Well-Being and International Sports Events," Journal of Economic Psychology *31, no. 2 (2010): 158-71.*
A Surprising Statistic
Mary C. Daly et al., "Dark Contrasts: The Paradox of High Rates of Suicide in Happy Places," Journal of Economic Behavior and Organization *80, no. 3 (2011): 435-42.*

10: The Downside of Happiness
There's More to Life Than Happiness
Jordi Quoidbach et al., "Emodiversity and the Emotional Ecosystem," Journal of Experimental Psychology: General *143, no. 6 (2014): 2057-66.*
Anthony D. Ong et al., "Emodiversity and Biomarkers of Inflammation," Emotion *(2017): https://doi.org/10.1037/emo0000343*
Mixed Emotions Boast Benefits
Jonathan M. Adler and Hal E. Hershfield, "Mixed Emotional Experience Is Associated with and Precedes Improvements in Psychological Well-Being," PLoS ONE *7, no. 4 (2012): e35633.*
Pursuing Happiness Can Make You Sad
Jonathan W. Schooler, Dan Ariely, and George Loewenstein, "The Pursuit and Assessment of Happiness Can Be Self-Defeating," The Psychology of Economic Decisions *1 (2003): 41-70.*
Iris B. Mauss et al., "Can Seeking Happiness Make People Unhappy? Paradoxical Effects of Valuing Happiness," Emotion *11, no. 4 (2011): 807-15.*
Pursuing Happiness Can Hurt Your Relationships
June Gruber, Iris B. Mauss, and Maya Tamir, "A Dark Side of Happiness? How, When, and Why Happiness Is Not Always Good," Perspectives on Psychological Science *6, no. 3 (2011): 222-33.*
Jill T. Levitt et al., "The Effects of Acceptance Versus Suppression of Emotion on Subjective and Psychophysiological Response to Carbon Dioxide Challenge in Patients with Panic Disorder," Behavior Therapy *35, no. 4 (2004): 747-66.*
Too Much Happiness Makes You . . .
Adam M. Grant and Barry Schwartz, "Too Much of a Good Thing: The Challenge and Opportunity of the Inverted U," Perspectives on Psychological Science, *6, no. 1 (2011): 61-76.*
. . . Take Too Many Risks
M. A. Cyders and G. T. Smith, "Emotion-Based Dispositions to Rash Action: Positive and Negative Urgency," Psychological Bulletin *134 (2008): 807-28.*
Howard S. Friedman et al., "Does Childhood Personality Predict Longevity?," Journal of Personality and Social Psychology *65, no. 1 (1993): 176-85.*
. . . Worse at Spotting Liars
Joseph P. Forgas and Rebekah East, "On Being Happy and Gullible: Mood Effects on Skepticism and the Detection of Deception," Journal of Experimental Social Psychology *44, no. 5 (2008): 1362-67.*

. . . Less Accurate

Lauren B. Alloy and Lyn Y. Abramson, "Judgment of Contingency in Depressed and Nondepressed Students: Sadder But Wiser?," Journal of Experimental Psychology: General 108, no. 4 (1979): 441–85.

. . . More Rigid

Barbara L. Fredrickson and Marcial F. Losada, "Positive Affect and the Complex Dynamics of Human Flourishing," American Psychologist 60, no. 7 (2005): 678–86.

. . . Less Creative

Mark A. Davis, "Understanding the Relationship Between Mood and Creativity: A Meta-Analysis," Organizational Behavior and Human Decision Processes 108, no. 1 (2009): 25–38.

. . . Psychopathic?

Richard P. Bentall, "A Proposal to Classify Happiness as a Psychiatric Disorder," Journal of Medical Ethics 18, no. 2 (1992): 94–98.

June Gruber, Iris B. Mauss, and Maya Tamir, "A Dark Side of Happiness? How, When, and Why Happiness Is Not Always Good," Perspectives on Psychological Science 6, no. 3 (2011): 222–33.

. . . Less Prepared to Fight or Flee

Gruber, Mauss, and Tamir, "A Dark Side of Happiness?"

. . . Selfish

Hui Bing Tan and Joseph P. Forgas, "When Happiness Makes Us Selfish, but Sadness Makes Us Fair: Affective Influences on Interpersonal Strategies in the Dictator Game," Journal of Experimental Social Psychology 46, no. 3 (2010): 571–76.

. . . Worse at Negotiating

Gerben A. Van Kleef, Carsten K. W. De Dreu, and Antony S. R. Manstead, "The Interpersonal Effects of Anger and Happiness in Negotiations," Journal of Personality and Social Psychology 86, no. 1 (2004): 57–76.

. . . Poorer and Less Educated

Shigehiro Oishi, Ed Diener, and Richard E. Lucas, "The Optimum Level of Well-Being: Can People Be Too Happy?," Perspectives on Psychological Science 2, no. 4 (2007): 346–60.

Getting Angry Has Its Perks

Maya Tamir and Brett Q. Ford, "Should People Pursue Feelings That Feel Good or Feelings That Do Good? Emotional Preferences and Well-Being," Emotion 12, no. 5 (2012): 1061–70.

What Doesn't Kill You . . .

Mark D. Seery, E. Alison Holman, and Roxane Cohen Silver, "Whatever Does Not Kill Us: Cumulative Lifetime Adversity, Vulnerability, and Resilience," Journal of Personality and Social Psychology 99, no. 6 (2010): 1025–41.

Don't Fake It

M. Frank, P. Ekman, and W. Friesen, "Behavioral Markers and Recognizability of the Smile of Enjoyment," Journal of Personality and Social Psychology 64, no. 1 (1993): 83–93.

Negative Is Smarter Than Positive

T. M. Amabile, "Brilliant but Cruel: Perceptions of Negative Evaluators," Journal of Experimental Social Psychology 19 (March 1983): 146–56.

Bad Is Stronger Than Good

R. F. Baumeister et al., "Bad Is Stronger Than Good," Review of General Psychology 5, no. 4 (2001): 323–70.

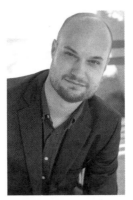

ABOUT THE AUTHOR

Alex Palmer is a journalist and excavator of fascinating facts. He is the *New York Times*–bestselling author of *The Santa Claus Man* as well as three other books of surprising bits of history and science: *Weird-o-Pedia*, *Alternative Facts*, and *Literary Miscellany*. His writing has appeared in *Lifehacker*, *Best Life*, *Mental Floss*, *Slate*, *Esquire*, and many other outlets.